Improving Surgical Skills and Outcomes

Stephen Lash

Improving Surgical Skills and Outcomes

A Multi-Perspective Approach

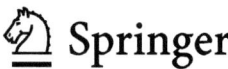 Springer

Stephen Lash
Southampton Eye Unit
University Hospital Southampton
Southampton, Hampshire, UK

ISBN 978-3-031-66689-6   ISBN 978-3-031-66690-2 (eBook)
https://doi.org/10.1007/978-3-031-66690-2

This Springer imprint is published by the registered company Springer Nature Switzerland AG
The registered company address is: Gewerbestrasse 11, 6330 Cham, Switzerland

If disposing of this product, please recycle the paper.

Yes Mr. Blackadder, How lucky I am that my job is also my hobby.
Blackadder 1989

The journey of surgery is long and arduous and it has not been possible without the support of my wonderful wife of over 25 years, Victoria. She tolerated my suggestions that I would 'Quite like to go back to University and study Medicine', to 'Train as a surgeon', to 'Do an MBA' and then to 'Go off to Australia with our three children for a year with a suitcase but nowhere to live!' I am also grateful to my children, Jonah, Abigail, Oscar and Esther for their support and tolerance of my often-long hours! Two are mad enough to try to follow me at the time of writing. And finally, all those who have given me their time and effort in training me, there are many. It's a privilege to be able to do this job and also great fun.

Foreword by Andrew Luff

Given the ever-expanding breadth of the medical school curriculum and volume of essential knowledge, it is no surprise that traditional medical training can be dominated by currently popular 'facts' and the science underpinning perceived good medical care. Having qualified in medicine in 1982 and spent the last 40 years of my working life in surgical specialties, I have witnessed the somewhat haphazard way we are taught (or, more frequently, not taught) the myriad of skills required to work safely, effectively and enjoyably as a surgeon.

Many patients tell me their job is a bit like mine, and they are probably right. Being a surgeon involves many skills, some obvious (a degree of manual dexterity is a big help) but others more nebulous, and less easy to acquire or perfect. We may be lucky enough to find a senior, or a contemporary, during our life-long learning who sees surgery as so much more than a technical exercise, bringing real meaning to what should be a beautiful art. This art must then be delivered in a cost-effective manner to an increasingly challenging health economy. Simultaneously, we hope to train the next generation of surgeons, learn from audit and contribute to research. All of this must be achieved remaining empathetic to our patients, colleagues and managers whilst (increasingly importantly) avoiding the disillusionment which threatens our profession.

In his book, Steve covers a variety of apparently disparate topics, which come together to help surgeons learn, operate safely, practice efficiently and teach. Once aware of these potentially neglected facets of our development I believe surgical trainers and educationalists will come to view these topics as core knowledge. As some of this may be completely new to the reader it might take time to assimilate and translate into real-world practice, but for each of us there may be gems which could improve care (for all patients, not just the ones currently in front of us) and enhance our working lives.

There are endless books about surgical technique, but a woeful lack of information on how to be a surgeon. This book helps fill that gap.

Prof. Andrew Luff, MA, MBBS,
FRCS, FRCOphth
Consultant Vitreoretinal Surgeon

Foreword by Giampaolo Gini

I first met Stephen Lash a few years ago during my time at Southampton University Hospital.

It did not take me long to become good friends with him and to realise that this was no ordinary individual I had come across.

As we sat each morning for a brief coffee break just before commencing a day's work, Steve would talk to me about his plans, ideas and aspirations … his eyes beaming with a contagious enthusiasm.

With time (and a growing addiction to coffee on my part) I began to understand Steve's unique and unconventional approach not only to the medical world but to life in general.

We found a common bond in an unwavering passion for surgery.

I do not use the word 'passion' lightly.

Passion is what keeps you up at night, mentally rehearsing the possible scenarios you will find in the next day's particularly complex case. It is the driving force which makes one look for innovative approaches to improve surgical and functional outcomes. It is what enables one to accept failure and learn from it.

Passion is what makes my every day in the operating theatre special and allows me to find gratification in solving a particularly challenging situation even after so many years of practice.

It is this passion which I try to instil in my fellows for I am convinced that this, not just the technicalities they learn, will make the difference in becoming a truly Great Surgeon.

This book is for anyone who is passionate about surgery, any branch of it.

It is divided into three main parts to simplify the presentation of the different topics but one can seamlessly glide from one box to the other.

Yet, I believe there is more to the book than making better surgeons.

As you read through its chapters you will see that you will not only be lead to thinking of ways in which you can improve your surgical skills but I believe you will also be challenged to consider other aspects of your everyday life and your personality.

Topics such as understanding one's reactions to stress (Individual Zones of Optimum Function).

Performance Mental Skills Training (PMST), individualised learning curves and Lean surgery are not only aimed at making you a technically better surgeon but can equally be applied to your everyday life experiences.

A chapter such as the one on 'Failure' and the concept of 'failing well' really goes beyond the realms of surgery and is an invitation for deeper reflection.

Equally compelling the one on 'Learning to Accept Responsibility' in a world where both in public life and in private relationships this concept is becoming obsolete.

In conclusion, a truly well-written and thoroughly thought-through book which synthesises the teachings learnt from many years of practice in the operating theatre.

I am convinced that it will not only appeal to the surgeons for which it was written but to a wider public as well.

After all what is an operating theatre if not an open window on the real world?

Giampaolo Gini, MD, Ph.D.
President of the European Vitreo
Retinal Society
Consultant Vitreo Retinal Surgeon
University Hospitals Sussex
Sussex, UK

Preface

It really did start over a coffee and surgical debrief after another busy list at the University Hospital Southampton where I had been a consultant ophthalmologist for over ten years. I had droned on about 'surfboards and confidence' and 'molehills and failing well' when my two fellows, Haytham Rezq and Mohamed Elnaggar, suggested I write a book about it all. So, I (eventually) did. The main aim of this book is to explore surgery from several diverse perspectives in the hope of shedding light on excellence and providing a potential road map to get there. It is aimed primarily at surgical trainees but I hope medical students and experienced surgeons will find it useful. It might even appeal to anyone interested in surgeons generally, a brief 'look behind the curtains'.

My plan of attack started with a (terrible) picture of a surgeon at a table in a theatre. I then drew three boxes, one around the table and hands, one around the surgeon's head and one that represented the theatre. With three boxes to boundary my thinking I populated them with possible topics and translated these thoughts into a Venn diagram. I began to see the overlaps, interactions and influences. I had a plan! The three boxes became the three parts to this book. I wanted to draw from outside medicine and give my own unique combination as an offering. There are books on aspects of what I cover but I wanted to bring a few novel perspectives together in one resource. This is not a technical manual of surgery; it is much deeper than that and I hope reveals the world behind the physical training. As such it will be useful to any surgeon in any sphere from the high street to the specialist unit. I suspect, as you read through, there will be moments of clarity in understanding why certain things are the way they are, as well as moments you gain new knowledge and hopefully, new enthusiasm to press on towards implementing it. I hope it will make all surgery even more interesting than it already is by exploring the immense complexity inherent in such an activity.

Writing it has enabled me to bring together major themes and interests in my life thus far. As a former optometrist I remember the feeling of being outside the surgical aspects of eye care and fascinated by it. How did surgeons even begin to perform surgery? After completing an MBA at the end of my surgical training I discovered new ways of thinking and looking at the world. I became more comfortable with

uncertainty and experimentation in thought and so when I finally began to perform surgery, I was obsessed with exploring what great looked like beyond the mechanics. Whenever I heard a consultant suggesting a trainee was a great surgeon I would ask why? Having 'good hands' was not enough detail for me. I even began to lead teaching sessions and give presentations as a new consultant on just this topic and so this book represents my finally scratching this particular itch, although not completely. In essence it's a book I wish I could have owned at the beginning of my training to inspire and direct me, enthuse and challenge me or at least, serve as an excellent conversation starter for the many 'coffee debriefs' I had as a trainee.
Enjoy

Southampton, UK   Stephen Lash

Acknowledgements

First and foremost, I must thank Haytham Rezq and Mohamed Elnaggar for encouraging me to write this book. It was not in my 5, 10 or any year plan and I am grateful for this left-field interruption, it has been great fun and a great challenge. I am grateful to my former teacher, mentor and now friend, Andy Luff for his input. He is a surgeon I have always looked up to (quite literally!) and having access to his immense brain and experience has been a great help and encouragement. He not only taught me much of what I know but he was also foremost in walking alongside me on this project with helpful suggestions as the book went back and forth by email with intermittent breakfast meetings to discuss progress. His foreword is gratefully received and much appreciated. I am grateful to Giampaolo Gini for agreeing to write a foreword. He is the most experienced surgeon I know having been around during the formative years of the profession and he still has enormous enthusiasm and energy for his surgery! He has been president of EVRS for many years and is well respected and well loved by all. I very much enjoyed working with him at Southampton for several years. I do not know what keeps him going! Thanks to Bernard Wolff, my South African fellow 'VR Fellow' in Melbourne and now close friend, for his input and criticism. He is also a deep thinker about these things and we have had many conversations over the years about all these topics! I am grateful to the airline pilot Captain David for giving me insight into their use of simulators but also an insight into the culture within the industry and their approach to problem solving and failure. If we could reproduce the airline culture in medicine it would look very different! I am grateful to Adrian Norton, former services and not medical at all, for reading it and giving his input and reassurance that it is an easy book to read and interesting, even to a non-medic. I am grateful to my wife, Victoria, for her support as I disappeared to write every week, she always has my back! Then there have been all the chance conversations and comments from people throughout my career who have in some way formed me and encouraged me, often without knowing it. Chris Canning, another mentor surgeon, for encouraging me to have something to aim for once more after a short lag post-failure. He is another deep thinker and efficient surgeon (now retired). Tom Williamson, not only for getting me the contact I needed to publish but also for his 'belt and braces' conversation at a conference over coffee that resulted in me beginning my journey into failing well. It's a team game for sure and we stand on the shoulders of those that have been there and done that and although there is nothing new under the sun, we sometimes need to learn to appreciate the rays once more. And finally, a big thanks to all my fellows who contributed not only to this book but to my education along the way. Teaching and training Specialist Trainees and Fellows is a privilege and I do not underestimate the value I obtain from doing it. They keep me sharp and curious and sometimes teach this old dog new tricks. There have been many but those who replied and bared their souls for the personality chapter were Amr Wasseff, Anthony Shinton, Chris Sinapis, Haytham Rezq, Mohammed El Naggar, Hassan Elkayal, Ben Clarke, Sandro De Simplicio, Abin Holla and Chee Kang. Thanks guys!

About This Book

The central quest of this book is, from C. S. Lewis, to 'Perambulate' in the fields of surgery. This book draws on my experiences as an eye surgeon over the last 23 years and especially over the last 13 years teaching and training junior surgeons. I will use three boxes to explore my key question, what makes a good surgeon and what makes them better. The perspectives are called boxes deliberately. It's good to think 'within' boxes, to extract all we can in the limited view permitted. It is also good to think 'outside the box'. However, when we think outside one box, we are simply thinking inside another, larger, less obvious one. I hope you will see how the boxes overlap and influence one another as you read on.

To grasp the structure of the book, picture a surgeon in theatre sitting at the table surrounded by staff and stuff, lights and laminar flow. Box 1 (explored in Part I) sits around the surgeon's hands. It is what is experienced in the surgical field in the moment of surgery. It is about dealing with stress and performing at the highest level, it is 'How' we do surgery. I will look at Sports Psychology and elite athletes and apply the techniques to surgery. I will look at airline pilots and explore simulators and assess their utility in our quest to becoming great surgeons and finally look at musicians and virtuosos and ask the question 'are we aiming high enough as surgeons?' Are there '*virtuosos*' in surgery or just '*primma donnas*'?

Box 2 (explored in Part II) sits around the surgeon's head and is the organisation and planning of surgery, it's the 'What' we do of surgery. I will explore Toyota car manufacturing and apply 'Lean' processes to surgery. Can we eliminate *muda* and pursue *Kaizen*? I also explore why we might not embrace 'Lean' looking at 'locus of control' and exploring 'failure' through the ages. Why is failure so hard and yet so useful and why is this the *worst* time in history to fail?

Box 3 (explored in Part III) is the theatre the surgeon is sitting in and the air they breathe. This is the least conscious of the three parts and asks the 'Why' of surgery. It explores decision making, heuristics and finally personality. It is perhaps the most powerful in terms of influence on the practice of surgery and yet the least seen, like the tiny rudder on a huge ship sitting beneath the surface.

Each part will be introduced with a fly over of the key themes and will be comprised of three chapters. Although there are many references, I am hoping the reader can forgo the need for an 'evidence base' and simply walk around in each perspective and see what might be of use in generating interesting thoughts, subsequent conversations and finally action. At the end of each chapter there will be some suggestions to try in order to apply the learnings. I am hoping the reader will own the paper book and take it with them to theatre, scribble all over it and spill coffee over it at the post-surgery debriefs. Surgery is physical. This book works better as a physical resource!

My hope is that in exploring surgery in these three parts anyone involved in surgery might benefit, from podiatry and dentistry on the high street to neurosurgery and ophthalmology in specialist units, from student to key opinion leader. I hope to stimulate ideas and thoughts and potential directions of travel that would lead the surgeon ever upward towards better surgery. It might also appeal to anyone interested in this particular breed of human willing to cut another in the pursuit of wholeness. Enjoy

2023   Stephen Lash

Contents

Part III The 'Why' of Surgery

About the Author

Stephen Lash BM, B.Sc. (Hons), MCOptom, FRCOphth, MBA

Consultant Ophthalmologist and Specialist in Vitreoretinal Surgery
University Hospital Southampton
Director/Surgeon- Lash Eye Care Ltd.
www.stephenlasheyesurgery.com

Stephen was born in Chatham in Kent on 5 November 1971 (The same year pars plana vitrectomy was born!) He studied for his BSc in Ophthalmic Optics at Aston University Birmingham from 1990–1993 and completed his pre-registration training at the Essex County Hospital in Colchester, Essex 1993–1994 with a prize for his professional examinations. It was during this year he met his wife, Victoria and applied and was accepted to study medicine at the University of Southampton. Following a year as a locum optometrist around Kent he was able to finance his studies and graduated in November 1999 with a prize for performance in medical finals and runner up two years in a row in the Duke Elder National Ophthalmology Examination. He was married to Victoria in 1998.

Stephen started ophthalmology training in 2001, following his house jobs at the University Hospital Southampton, as an SHO in Bournemouth. He gained a position on the Wessex rotation in ophthalmology completing this in 2009. For the last 18 months of his rotation, he completed an executive MBA part-time at the University of Southampton Management School and was awarded the prize for the top mark in his year. He then went to Australia for a fellowship in VR surgery at the Royal Victorian Eye and Ear Hospital, Melbourne, with his wife and three children, Jonah, Abigail and Oscar. Following this intensive year, he returned as a Locum consultant to the University Hospital Southampton in 2010 and was appointed to his substantive post in 2011. Esther came along in 2011 to complete the family although having the older two move out to do medicine at Manchester and Birmingham the family have now acquired a Golden retriever, Monty. He continues to work part-time as an NHS consultant in Southampton and is passionate about training and education. He is also a director of Lash Eye Care and provides private care as well as education for local optometrists, trainees and fellow consultants.

Outside of work, Stephen provides mentoring for students from his local church, enjoys walking, red wine, coffee, learning about culture, philosophy, theology and anything really now family life is increasingly less busy! He is very physically active, even after his hip replacement, regularly cycling and swimming in an attempt to battle anno domini, a fight he will lose. This is his first book.

Part I
The 'How' of Surgery

Introduction

'Part I' will explore the 'How' of surgery and what might improve performance both in the '*preparation for*' and in the '*moment of*' surgery. As I hope you will see as you read through the various 'boxes', this represents a very limited view of surgery and yet performance in this 'box' often draws the most attention and judgement. "They have good hands!"

The cornerstone chapter will focus on Sports Psychology and how it might usefully be applied to the practice of surgery and further, how Sports Psychology might contribute to continual improvement. The next chapter will explore the obvious tool for improving surgery, other than the patient, the surgical simulator. I will draw comparisons with airline pilots and assess the utility of simulators with reference to 'learning curves'—whatever they are! I will move from elite athletes to musical virtuosos, examining aspects of musical performance and practice. What does it take to become a concert pianist? What might 'surgical virtuosity' look like and can it even be achieved? Finally, I will draw together the findings and argue for a shift in the paradigm of performance that might encourage progress. Are we aiming high enough as surgeons? Striving for Virtuosity or surviving as prima donnas?

Caveat

I will provide an evidence base for my thoughts although, and you may struggle with this, this is not my highest priority. When I started my MBA, I remember discussing with one of the professors that intellectually, I was used to walking around in shoes on concrete and the MBA felt more like strolling in the sand barefoot and I was finding it a struggle. If you are used to intellectual wanderings on concrete, I invite you remove your shoes and explore the sands. I have often struggled with the paradigm of evidence-based medicine in such a performative arena as surgery-'yes, but what about in *my* hands?' However, as a surgeon or 'surgeon to be' reading this, I will assume you are expecting at least a board walk through the sand but my real hope for you is to be found well beyond. I hope to generate ideas and thoughts, provide some challenges and new perspectives but also suggest some practical applications to aid your performance. Although my experience is within the field of ophthalmology and many examples will be drawn from this, I hope the concepts explored will be applicable to all surgical fields from the high street to specialist hospitals. It is a journey I am on with you and I will share my own personal experiences, triumphs and failures!

Chapter 1
Sports Psychology—What Can We Learn from Elite Athletes?

Confidence is great. If you have it you can share it; if you don't, you can borrow it. But ideally, you need to acquire it for yourself.
—Stephen Lash

In surgery, the past stretches back and the future stretches forward, but the present is a razor-sharp scalpel you must balance on. It only cuts if you slip off.
—Stephen Lash

Abstract I will explore what Sports Psychology has to offer because it deals with the reactions and responses to stress and their effect on performance under pressure but also how to prepare to perform at your best. There is an increasing interest in applying Sports Psychology techniques to healthcare (Sandars et al. Sandars et al., Med Teach 44:71–78, 2022). Surgery involves making many decisions, often under pressure, often with uncertain outcomes, in an ever-changing surgical environment, and this results in a degree of stress felt in the body and the mind. Some stress can be helpful but too much can result in a failure to perform or even 'Catastrophe'. Pressure can come externally from the need to deliver high volumes, complexity of cases, complications, theatre environment, bureaucracy and the team as well as internally with the fear of failure ranking highly. I will explore 'failure' in 'Part II'. Character traits and personality might also play a role although and I will explore these in 'Part III'.

Keywords Sports psychology · Surgical decision-making · Catastrophe model · Goal setting theory · Surgeon's performance

1.1 Stress and Performance

We have all been there, and if you are not yet a surgeon, you will be going there so buckle up. The case was meant to be straightforward but is rapidly spiralling out of control (usually y*our own* fault). The end of the theatre session approaches and the next team are waiting. An emergency has just walked through the door. Your critical boss is peering at you with a questioning look on their face or your trainee is rapidly losing their unrealistic opinion of you. Your trainee has just done something surprising and sudden; you have just done something stupid and are now in a hole, perhaps rapidly filling with blood. You look around for someone to blame and catch your own reflection in the monitor screen and think better of it. Surgery is about making many decisions under varying degrees of stress and it can go from utter apparent 'control' and witty banter with the team to chaos and silence. How does stress effect performance and what can we do about it anyway?

1.2 The Catastrophe Model (Hardy 1987)

The Catastrophe model represents a theory which attempts to predict the interactive effects of cognitive anxiety (fear of failure), physiological arousal (increased heart rate and sweating) and performance (Fig. 1.1). Imagine Fig. 1.1 is a view into a room with an odd-shaped curved ceiling, solid back and side walls but no front wall. Now imagine (or remember) you are the trainee working with a very competent and understanding boss on a case you are familiar with. A little fear of failure is good, you are keen to impress, but you know nothing can really go wrong with '*them*' there. This is the 'back wall' of Fig. 1.1. You 'borrow' their confidence and your cognitive anxiety is very low. When cognitive anxiety is low, physiological arousal has an inverted 'U' shape with increasing performance up to a peak and then deteriorating performance thereafter but it is a subtle decline. As the case progresses there are minor deviations and stresses but this increased arousal focusses the mind and improves your performance and anyway, you know the boss is there. I would argue that this is exactly the environment needed for the new surgeon, and it is the responsibility of the boss to provide this although there are bosses who cannot provide this given their own attitude to risk and failure which I will explore in 'Part III'. A surgical simulator can also provide just such a scenario. Anyway, your boss is so pleased with your progress that they nip off for a coffee and let you get on with it. The case starts to go '*off Piste*'. Cognitive anxiety skyrockets, you are on your own. You rapidly move away from the safety of the 'back wall' towards the front of the room, and with increasing physiological arousal your performance suddenly plummets, you lose it, you fall apart. When cognitive anxiety is high, an increased level of physiological arousal beyond a certain 'tipping point' leads to a catastrophic reduction in performance. Unfortunately, the reality is that we all need to experience both scenarios in order to progress as surgeons. Complete control is an illusion and who does not fear failure?

From my experience as a surgeon this model makes intuitive sense. Most experienced surgeons are likely to have low levels of physiological arousal and cognitive anxiety. They are very comfortable in most situations, having experienced them over time, and have multiple options available to them as cases become complex and further, most surgeons score low in trait neuroticism on the 'Big 5 Factor' model of personality. I will explore this in 'Part III'. I have experienced the 'collapse' and

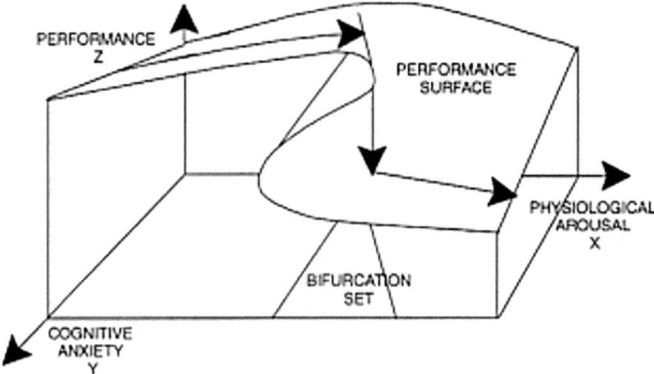

Fig. 1.1 Originally included in 'The Inverted-U Hypothesis: A Catastrophe for Sport Psychology', John Fazey, Lew Hardy, British Association of Sports Sciences and the National Coaching Foundation, 1988. Reproduced by kind permission of UK Coaching (Formerly National Coaching foundation)

it is unpleasant. Thought processes start to reach into the future and consequences flood in distracting me from the present moment. Adrenaline release interferes with fine motor control and decision making. In this state, movements get clumsy and thought processes cloudy. This model is useful to explain these experiences but it also provides some targets for intervention, notably controlling physiological arousal and techniques to reduce cognitive anxiety.

1.3   Individual Zones of Optimum Function (IZOF)—'in the Zone!'

However, the correlation proposed in the Catastrophe model may be more nuanced in individuals. In his theory of Individual Zones of Optimum Function (IZOF), Hanin proposed that each athlete (performer) has a specific zone of optimal function and this may be at low, medium or high anxiety levels. Provided the athlete performs within their IZOF they will perform at an optimal level (Hanin 1995). The zones of the athletes were determined after completing a detailed Standardised Emotional Scale and assessment. Although detailed assessment may be useful for individual surgeons (if you are really keen!), it is well worth one simply being aware of previous situations and the levels of stress, emotional responses and resultant performance to gain some insight into where your zone might be and also to understand that others (trainees/consultants) might perform optimally in a different zone.

For example, I am aware that I perform best when there is Friday afternoon NHS list with lots of emergencies added on and the team are motivated to finish on time. Pace and turnover are optimal for me at this level of stress. However, a list starting an hour late with a very slow turnaround is my worst nightmare. My trainees and staff have suggested that I am like a puppy who needs something to amuse himself with as I pace up and down trying to do something, anything! In this state surgery does not flow, I may be prone to over thinking and over intervening. I wonder if a surgeons' IZOF subtly determines which specialty they go into or even whether they become a surgeon in the first place? Perhaps we naturally veer towards a good match, in terms of stress, between and even within specialities?

1.4   Stress in the Surgical Arena—The Evidence

In a review of the impact of surgical stress on performance, Arora identified that pressure results in physical, mental and physiological arousal. Although performance is initially enhanced at lower levels of arousal, consistent with the Catastrophe model, at higher levels performance suffers both physically, with impaired motor function, but perhaps more significantly, with cognitive effects resulting in shifts in decision making (Arora et al. 2010). These effects seem to be moderated by experience, again consistent with the Catastrophe model with lower levels of cognitive anxiety likely present in more experienced surgeons. In another study of 16 surgeons, a wide range of intraoperative stressors were identified. Although some stress was seen as positive, undue levels of stress impaired judgement, decision making, communication and teamwork (Wetzel et al. 2006). This study also demonstrated that senior surgeons had coping mechanisms to deal with the undue stress as opposed to the more junior surgeons.

In another study, Anton surveyed surgeons' triggers and responses to 9 stressors on operative performance. Seventy-two responses were received. The highest stresses were associated with complex or rarely performed cases and poor assistance (I would like to come back to *this* particular finding in 'Part II' with the concept of 'locus of control'). 40% of surgeons indicated that they had witnessed an intraoperative complication directly related to surgeon stress. Surgeons used a variety of techniques to deal with stress but 82% believed that formal stress management training would be beneficial (Anton et al. 2015).

Looking specifically at decision making under stress, Wemm found that men tended to become more risk preferring under stress in a linear fashion, ignoring potential consequences of their decisions, and this correlated with increasing heart rates. Women were more conservative up to a certain level of stress but beyond this, decision making deteriorated in a more curvilinear fashion (Wemm and Wulfert 2017).

A technique I find useful is inspired by Sun Tzu in his book 'Art of War' published in 401. 'When you arrive on enemy land, burn your boats' (Sun Tzu 2007). When you arrive at a complication the only way is forward, keep calm and keep going, your back is against the wall. I must admit that this approach may be more appropriate with experience and might drift into arrogance if applied too early on in your career! I also become more risk preferring under stress but this is partly related to my personality which we explore in 'Part III'.

1.5   Interventions

Interventions should ideally reduce cognitive anxiety and physiological arousal. In reality I am not sure I have met a surgeon who performs at their best when everything is falling apart and stress levels are high unlike the athlete who uses this energy, aggression and fear to triumph. The literature agrees and does suggest that high levels of physiological arousal and cognitive anxiety are associated with poor performance in surgery and so interventions would need to reduce them both rather than ramp them up! The interventions should facilitate good cognitive function allowing good decision making, communication and teamwork and reduce the physiological effects of stress likely to impair fine motor control.

1.6   Performance Mental Skills Training (PMST)

Vealey suggested that the term Performance Mental Skills Training (PMST) should 'describe specific cognitive and behavioural skills for maintaining optimal mental arousal, physical arousal, and attention immediately before and during a challenging situation'. (Vealey 1988) This is not to say good mental health hygiene and calm preparation are not important but I want to focus on the moment of surgery in 'Part I'.

   Anton reviewed the effectiveness of PMST in surgery and looked at several key areas including mental imagery, energy management, attention and thought management, goal setting and performance routines. (Anton et al. 2017) I will explore each in turn and, having reviewed the evidence, look at personal and practical examples and applications.

1.7   Mental Imagery

Mental imagery is defined as a 'mental simulation process which allows a person to represent a perceptual, multisensory scenario in their mind, without any actual sensory input' (Munzert et al. 2009). It has to be *multi*sensory and in very fine detail to be effective. Jeannerod's simulation theory, that 'common cortical motor systems are activated when imaging, observing or executing an action', provides the scientific basis for this form of cognitive training (Jeannerod 2001). Imagery has also been explored using functional imaging demonstrating that similar neural pathways are activated during cognitive training as in physical training (Seiler et al. 2015). Furthermore, a study by Debarnot found that the brain changes resulting from cognitive training for specific motor tasks mimic those observed after physical practice (Debarnot et al. 2014). 'Thinking' seems to be as powerful as 'doing' in neuroplasticity terms which is quite incredible. Mental imagery is the most widely researched mental skill in performance psychology and has been shown to be effective in enhancing performance in athletes and musicians and even developing motor skills during rehabilitation (Cicerone et al. 2011; Schinke et al. 2016). However, imagery is limited to tasks previously performed. One can only truly imagine what one has actually performed (Mulla et al. 2012).

Imagery involves engaging the imagination by going through the actions in detail in the mind and this should be as 'real life' as possible hence the need to have actually performed the tasks in the real world. The literature is rather vague on what is actually required of subjects. Arora provided excellent detail in their study in terms of the script used. For example, 'use the diathermy to dissect the fatty tissue', becomes 'You gently touch the fat with the heel of the diathermy and can hear a buzzing noise. As you do so, smoke begins to fill the abdomen…' (Arora et al. 2011) Hall explored the potential role for imagery during the acquisition of surgical skills and found that it helped surgeons better understand the steps of a procedure, reduced the learning curve, facilitated the transfer of skills to a novel but related technique, limited decay of skills and optimised preparation for a complex procedure (Hall 2002). Several other RCTs have also investigated the role of imagery. Arora demonstrated that during simulated cholecystectomy those that received imagery training significantly outperformed controls that had received physical practice alone. (Arora et al. 2011).

It is interesting to note, given the consequences explored in the Catastrophe model, that frequently participants felt better prepared, less stressed and better able to perform the task regardless of the actual benefit, or not, of mental imagery. Methodology between studies was very variable as were the subjects which included medical students and surgeons. Intervention and outcome measures also differed with both simulated and real scenarios assessed (Sandars et al. 2022b). Wallace reviewed the studies specific to surgical education that had a positive and a negative effect and found key differences that might explain the results. Positive effect studies involved longer and more repetitive sessions of mental rehearsal than those in the negative group. Not only were they at least 30 min long they were also delivered by trained 'cognitive trainers' or experienced psychologists using very structured mental processes multiple times (Wallace et al. 2017).

From my own experience I believe it is worthwhile even in the absence of trained professionals. I have certainly found it very useful. On long train journeys to distant hospitals on my junior surgical rotation I would sit and think in detail about surgery, losing myself in this 'other world'. I would plan a surgery, introduce a specific complication and then manage it, over and over again in my mind. I would get the adrenaline rush of real life. When I eventually had the specific complication in real life it did not feel so unfamiliar and I was able to proceed with much less stress. However, when I have used imagery to visualise a novel technique or even an extension to an existing technique, I have noticed, with significant frustration, that it never goes quite the way I had imagined in the moment of surgery. It is then I am reminded of the military quote attributed to Helmuth von Moltke in 1871—'No plan of operations extends with any certainty beyond the first encounter with the main enemy forces'. Although I believe imagery can be of use, it cannot be an occasional fleeting thought but rather an obsession! One has to delve deep and often and it has to be surgical techniques you have actually performed.

1.8 Energy Management

Energy management skills help to regulate physiological arousal which has been identified as one of the significant factors in terms of impacting physical performance. One of the best methods to reduce the effects of this stress is to control the breathing, especially deep, rhythmic, diaphragmatic breathing to counter the shallow breathing encountered under stress. Deep, diaphragmatic breathing has been shown to increase vagal tone and stimulate the parasympathetic system counteracting the sympathetic fight or flight response in stressful situations (Magnon et al. 2021). Increasing parasympathetic tone is also likely to have an effect on reducing tremor, which in itself can reduce stress for a surgeon, improving surgical manoeuvres.

I tend to use deep breathing in certain situations which require very fine motor control as well as sitting back and breathing when I find myself in a complicated situation. I like to make progress at all times but sometimes the best way to make progress (in the right direction) is to stop, breathe and think.

1.9 Attention/Thought Management

Concentration is critical in elite sports and in surgery. Selective attention on the task requires the screening out of distracting or irrelevant stimuli, one needs to be completely in the moment. These distracting stimuli can come from the external environment, from background chatter, distracting music and even from teaching and training. These external sources are perhaps easier to control than the internal sources of distraction, stress, anxiety and negative thoughts. Where the cognitive–affective domain is involved, responses may show as negative thoughts, uncontrolled cognitions, disruptions of attention or concentration, worry, dread or hypervigilance (Suinn 2005). There are a variety of interventions for these unhelpful thoughts and include cognitive restructuring (confronting the irrationality of the thoughts and restructuring them to match reality), positive thought control (replacing negative thoughts with positive self-instruction), thought isolation (taking the negative thought and stopping it, perhaps by picturing a large stop sign) and attentional refocussing (attending to non-stressful stimuli) (Suinn 2005). Evidence of benefit within surgery is limited. Maher found a trend towards improved performance in year one and three surgical residents with training in energy and attention management and imagery. Despite only a 'trend' in actual improved performance, 91% of respondents found the training valuable (Maher et al. 2013). One aspect we will discuss in 'Part III' may have a powerful effect on attention and energy management, notably System 1 versus System 2 operation. As a result, care also has to be taken when training as discussing 'in the moment' with a trainee mid-surgery can result in distraction for them. It is usually better to do this at debrief over coffee.

Most of the time I am very relaxed about background noise in the theatre. I like to play background music to cover up the medical noises of pulse oximeters, and talk to the patient throughout surgery—they are under local anaesthetic by the way. Talking relaxes me and the patient as does humour (I do try). However, there are certain times when I have to specifically focus and at these times chatter and music can be a distraction. I know I am out of my IZOF or perhaps 'flow state' when I become too aware of what is going on around me and drift out of the present moment. I am not alone. Allen and Blascovich studied the autonomic responses and performance of surgeons under several conditions; silence, investigator-selected music (Pachelbel's Canon in D) and self-selected music. Autonomic reactivity was significantly reduced in the surgeon-selected music category followed by investigator selected music then silence. Speed and accuracy of movements were also best in self-selected music and worst in silence (Allen 1994). However, another study found that when it came to complex manoeuvres, music made no difference suggesting the surgeon could block out noise, including music, with the intense concentration required for such manoeuvres (Moorthy et al. 2004). Music in theatre may also improve performance of the team as well as the surgeon. In one study, 63% of professionals considered that music in theatre had a positive effect on communication and nearly 80% believed that music made people calmer and more efficient (Ullmann et al. 2008).

1.10   Goal Setting Theory

Goal setting theory attempts to explain the relationship between goals and task performance. It is a motivational theory of human behaviour and relies on goals having several moderators including difficulty, specificity and time orientation (Tosi et al. 1991). I find this is a very important and useful tool and it maybe it you too have already, unknowingly, been doing this for years. It makes intuitive sense. It encourages the athlete to break down the task into a series of smaller tasks. Perfection can be determined and visualised and then an attempt to match this is performed and then mentally graded before moving onto the next task. Surgically, I have called these the 'mini-games' that I play. This fits very well into 'Lean' in 'Part II' and is also likely to result in marginal gains which are important in improving performance in any sphere, including surgery. It also facilitates imagery as you are forced to micro-dissect your actions into micro-technique for the specific task, enriching the detail to be used in imagery. My goals include achieving an intention to execution ratio of 1:1, with each manoeuvre right first time with minimal movement and minimal time wasted. I determine what perfect looks like for each particular section of my surgery, and although I never achieve a perfect score in all tasks, I may get close in some. Because I am driven to focus on achieving a perfect score in each step, this goal draws me into each isolated present moment. I also get to mentally rehearse each task before I complete it.

1.11   Performance Routines

Performance routines are frequently seen in sports, Jonny Wilkinson comes to mind. The routines bring to the forefront of the mind the subsequent actions required, focussing attention and moderating physiological arousal (Cotterill 2010). This fits very well with goal setting theory.

On reflection I have several of these, from holding the Iodine during the team brief to how I prepare to peel layers off the retina to things I say to the patient. Familiarity reduces stress and I encourage my trainees to do things the same way every time to build this muscle memory, to push the control to the brain stem, to operate in 'System 1'which I will discuss in 'Part III'. This strategy frees up mental capacity to make decisions and spot potential threats to progress.

Having explored each technique in detail, the evidence is generally derived from combinations of these techniques and it is in the combination that Elite Athletes benefit. I can see how these techniques would be embraced by the highly driven athlete whose performance is survival and how the infrastructure in Elite sport would facilitate it through training and resources. What about surgeons working in complex organisations with limited funding and resources?

1.12   Does Performance Mental Skills Training (PMST) Actually Work in Surgery?

McDonald conducted in-depth interviews with 33 highly proficient surgeons using a framework based on Orlick's 'Model of Human Excellence' which puts commitment and belief at the heart of the 'Wheel of Excellence' with peripheral domains of positive images, mental readiness, full focus, distraction control and constructive evaluation (Orlick and Partington 1988). Of the three major readiness factors rated by the surgeons, mental, technical, and physical, surgeons rated mental readiness as the most important for performance excellence in surgery *above* technical and physical readiness (McDonald et al. 1995). These included commitment, self-belief, positive imagery, mental readiness, full focus, distraction control and constructive evaluation.

A review of 20 studies by Sanders et al. suggested that PMST was potentially effective for surgeons but that the training was complex, multifaceted and implemented in very different ways in the studies (Sandars et al. 2022a). The majority of studies used mental imagery ($n = 19$) with relaxation ($n = 12$), self-talk ($n = 12$) and goal setting ($n = 8$), especially in combination ($n = 13$). They found that combining imagery, self-talk and relaxation delivered face to face by an experienced trainer over five sessions of 57-min duration was associated with significant positive outcomes. However, the review highlights the difficulties in the methods of application with each technique, how the measurements were made and the outcomes determined between studies. Closed clinical scenarios were static, stable and predictable whereas as open clinical skills were performed in real-life scenarios with added complexity and so very difficult to compare (Sandars et al. 2022a). Anton also conducted a review of 28 papers and found that although the majority of the literature suggests that mental imagery and stress management training programmes were effective at enhancing surgical performance and reducing stress, studies from other disciplines suggested that comprehensive mental skills programmes may be more effective than imagery and stress management techniques alone (Anton et al. 2017). Stefanidis looked at the effectiveness of a mental skills curriculum in enhancing surgical performance with a group of 55 participants. Compared to controls the intervention group significantly improved their mental skill use, demonstrated higher laparoscopic skill improvement during retention (although this was a small effect) and reported less stress during the transfer test from simulator to porcine models (Stefanidis et al. 2017).

1.13 Sport Versus Medicine

Von Guenthner implemented weekly mental skills training sessions with six elite cross-country skiers which included goal setting, imagery, energy management, attention management, confidence, motivation and performance routines (Guenthner 2010). All participants improved in goal setting, 83% improved in self-talk, relaxation and imagery scores whilst reducing their anxiety, 67% improved in emotional control and self-confidence and 50% improved their attentional control and all rated the effectiveness of the programme highly. The programme lasted one year, divided into four cycles and was intense.

In the medical setting, Aronson assessed the impact of mental skills training on stress responses in simulated resuscitations and also the residents' perceptions of this intervention (Aronson et al. 2022). They used the 'Breath, Talk, See, Focus' (BTSF) mental performance tool. Breathe: 'box breathing' to reduce physiological stress; Talk: Positive self-talk, recited with intention and repeated frequently; See: Visualisation of successful completion of a task; Focus: Use of a cue word to turn on selective attention. Preparation involved a 20-min didactic lecture one month before the activity but participants were encouraged to practice using the tool during their normal work. The study found no difference in objective or subjective stress measures although, again, participants found the training useful.

I think one can appreciate the vastly differing resources that went into the skiers and the medics, this is surely not surprising. It is easier to deliver this training to an extremely motivated, small group of rare individuals as opposed to a large cohort of surgeons both practically and economically.

1.14 Conclusion

Although I do not think we can match the intensity of PMST for Elite athletes in medicine I still believe it can be of benefit to the enthusiastic surgeon. From the studies, mental imagery is the most important followed by relaxation, self-talk and goal setting. However, it is up to the individual surgeon to embrace these techniques and practice them in their own time. I have certainly found them very useful in my own surgery especially imagery and goal setting and these have augmented my approach to 'Lean' surgery which I will discuss in 'Part II'.

1.15 To Try

1.15.1 Catastrophe Model

Does this ring true in your experience?

Have you had the collapse and if so, what happened?

Do you borrow your trainer's confidence and if so, how can you build your own?

1.15.2 IZOF

Where is your zone? Reflect on a task that went really well and what the level of physiological arousal was at the time, do you ever feel in the zone? Can you replicate this ensuring lists are booked appropriately and run at a level of efficiency consistent with your IZOF. Consider getting evaluated if you are really keen.

1.15.3 Imagery

Consider how you can introduce this PMS technique into your training. Try mental imagery but remember you need absolute detail in every sense, you must feel the tension and adrenaline and you must have performed what you are imaging in the real world.

1.15.4   Attention Management

Can you improve the environment in theatre to boost performance (Music?).

How do you deal with negative thoughts during surgery, can you distract, refocus, reframe?

1.15.5   Goal Setting

Can you split surgery into many small parts or mini-games? Having done this, decide what a score of 100% would look like and then compare your performance after each 'mini-game'. How well did you do, what could be better? Can you refine what 100% looks like? Repeat for each 'mini-game' and so on. But review each section as you go- do not rely on annual Audit!

Consider recording your surgery, if at all possible, and reviewing the 'mini-games' at a later time with a senior surgeon.

1.15.6   Performance Routines

Can you develop performance routines or recognise you already have them? How can they help you to prepare for what follows?

1.15.7   Energy Management

Be aware of physiological arousal during surgery and try to moderate it using breathing techniques. Does it work?

References

Allen K. Effects of music on cardiovascular reactivity among surgeons. JAMA: J Am Med Ass. 1994;272(11):882. https://doi.org/10.1001/jama.1994.03520110062030

Anton NE, Montero PN, Howley LD, Brown C, Stefanidis D. What stress coping strategies are surgeons relying upon during surgery? Am J Surgery. 2015;210(5):846–51. https://doi.org/10.1016/j.amjsurg.2015.04.002.

Anton NE, Bean EA, Hammonds SC, Stefanidis D. Application of mental skills training in surgery: A review of its effectiveness and proposed next steps. J Laparoendoscopic Adv Surg Tech. 2017;27(5):459–469. Mary Ann Liebert Inc. https://doi.org/10.1089/lap.2016.0656

Aronson M, Henderson T, Dodd K, Cirone M, Putman M, Salzman D, Lovell E, Williamson K. Effects of brief mental skills training on emergency medicine residents' stress response during a simulated resuscitation: a prospective randomized trial. Western J Emer Med. 2022;23(1):79–85. https://doi.org/10.5811/westjem.2021.10.53892.

Arora S, Sevdalis N, Nestel D, Woloshynowych M, Darzi A, Kneebone R. The impact of stress on surgical performance: a systematic review of the literature. Surgery. 2010;147(3):318-330.e6. https://doi.org/10.1016/j.surg.2009.10.007.

Arora S, Aggarwal R, Sirimanna P, Moran A, Grantcharov T, Kneebone R, Sevdalis N, Darzi A. Mental practice enhances surgical technical skills. Ann Surg. 2011;253(2):265–70. https://doi.org/10.1097/SLA.0b013e318207a789.

Cicerone KD, Langenbahn DM, Braden C, Malec JF, Kalmar K, Fraas M, Felicetti T, Laatsch L, Harley JP, Bergquist T, Azulay J, Cantor J, Ashman T. Evidence-based cognitive rehabilitation: updated review of the literature from 2003 through 2008. Arch Phys Med Rehabil. 2011;92(4):519–30. https://doi.org/10.1016/j.apmr.2010.11.015.

Cotterill S. Pre-performance routines in sport: current understanding and future directions. Int Rev Sport Exerc Psychol. 2010;3(2):132–53. https://doi.org/10.1080/1750984X.2010.488269.

Debarnot U, Sperduti M, di Rienzo F, Guillot A. Experts bodies, experts minds: how physical and mental training shape the brain. Front Human Neurosc 2014;8. https://doi.org/10.3389/fnhum.2014.00280

Guenthner SHJBDKL. Smoke and mirrors or wave of the future? Evaluating a mental skills training program for elite cross-country skiers. J Sport Behavior. 2010;33:3–24.

Hall JC. Imagery practice and the development of surgical skills. Am J Surgery. 2002;184(5):465–70. https://doi.org/10.1016/S0002-9610(02)01007-3.

Hanin, Y. (1995). Individual zones of optimal functioning (IZOF) model: an idiographicapproach to performance anxiety. Sport psychology: an analysis of athletebehavior (Third). Mouvement Publications.

Hardy L, FJ. The inverted U hypothesis: a catastrophe for sport psychology. The annual conference of the north American society for the psychology for sport and physical activity 1987.

Jeannerod M. Neural simulation of action: a unifying mechanism for motor cognition. Neuroimage. 2001;14(1):S103–9. https://doi.org/10.1006/nimg.2001.0832.

Magnon V, Dutheil F, Vallet GT. Benefits from one session of deep and slow breathing on vagal tone and anxiety in young and older adults. Sci Rep. 2021;11(1):19267. https://doi.org/10.1038/s41598-021-98736-9.

Maher Z, Milner R, Cripe J, Gaughan J, Fish J, Goldberg AJ. Stress training for the surgical resident. Am J Surgery. 2013;205(2):169–74. https://doi.org/10.1016/j.amjsurg.2012.10.007.

McDonald J, Orlick T, Letts M. Mental readiness in surgeons and its links to performance excellence in surgery. J Pediatric Orthopaed. 1995;15(5):691–7. https://doi.org/10.1097/01241398-199509000-00027.

Moorthy K, Munz Y, Undre S, Darzi A. Objective evaluation of the effect of noise on the performance of a complex laparoscopic task. Surgery. 2004;136(1):25–30. https://doi.org/10.1016/j.surg.2003.12.011.

Mulla M, Sharma D, Moghul M, Kailani O, Dockery J, Ayis S, Grange P. Learning basic laparoscopic skills: a randomized controlled study comparing box trainer, virtual reality simulator, and mental training. J Surg Educ. 2012;69(2):190–5. https://doi.org/10.1016/j.jsurg.2011.07.011.

Munzert J, Lorey B, Zentgraf K. Cognitive motor processes: the role of motor imagery in the study of motor representations. Brain Res Rev. 2009;60(2):306–26. https://doi.org/10.1016/j.brainresrev.2008.12.024.

Orlick T, Partington J. Mental links to excellence. The Sport Psychol. 1988;2(2):105–30. https://doi.org/10.1123/tsp.2.2.105.

Rufai SR, Mitchell BG, Farmer TD, Lash SC. Reducing anxiety during conscious surgery—a patient survey. Int J Surg. 2015;23:118–9. https://doi.org/10.1016/j.ijsu.2015.09.058.

Sandars J, Jenkins L, Church H, Patel R, Rumbold J, Maden M, Patel M, Henshaw K, Brown J. Applying sport psychology in health professions education: a systematic review of performance mental skills training. Med Teach. 2022;44(1):71–8. https://doi.org/10.1080/0142159X.2021.1966403.

Schinke RJ, McGannon KR, Smith B (Eds) (2016) Routledge international handbook of sport psychology. Routledge. https://doi.org/10.4324/9781315777054

Seiler BD, Monsma EV, Newman-Norlund RD. Biological evidence of imagery abilities: intraindividual differences. J Sport and Exerc Psychol. 2015;37(4):421–35. https://doi.org/10.1123/jsep.2014-0303.

Stefanidis D, Anton NE, Howley LD, Bean E, Yurco A, Pimentel ME, Davis CK. Effectiveness of a comprehensive mental skills curriculum in enhancing surgical performance: results of a randomized controlled trial. Am J Surgery. 2017;213(2):318–24. https://doi.org/10.1016/j.amjsurg.2016.10.016.

Suinn RM. Behavioral intervention for stress management in sports. Int J Stress Manag. 2005;12(4):343–62. https://doi.org/10.1037/1072-5245.12.4.343.

Tosi HL, Locke EA, Latham GP. A theory of goal setting and task performance. Acad Manag Rev. 1991;16(2):480. https://doi.org/10.2307/258875.

Tzu S (2007) The art of war. Harper Press

Ullmann Y, Fodor L, Schwarzberg I, Carmi N, Ullmann A, Ramon Y. The sounds of music in the operating room. Injury. 2008;39(5):592–7. https://doi.org/10.1016/j.injury.2006.06.021.

Vealey RS. Future directions in psychological skills training. The Sport Psychol. 1988;2(4):318–36.

Wallace L, Raison N, Ghumman F, Moran A, Dasgupta P, Ahmed K. Cognitive training: how can it be adapted for surgical education? The Surgeon. 2017;15(4):231–9. https://doi.org/10.1016/j.surge.2016.08.003.

Wemm SE, Wulfert E. Effects of acute stress on decision making. Appl Psychophysiol Biofeedback. 2017;42(1):1–12. https://doi.org/10.1007/s10484-016-9347-8.

Wetzel CM, Kneebone RL, Woloshynowych M, Nestel D, Moorthy K, Kidd J, Darzi A. The effects of stress on surgical performance. Am J Surg. 2006;191(1):5–10. https://doi.org/10.1016/j.amjsurg.2005.08.034.

Chapter 2
Surgical Simulators—What Can We Learn from Pilots?

There are no surgical hacks and no magic- just slow, deliberate formation in the direction of excellence. So, you'd better have an idea of what excellence looks like and take every opportunity to achieve it.

—Stephen Lash

We seem to prefer the views from the foothills of the learning curve. The views from the peak are much better, but require an awful lot of time and effort to reach.

—Stephen Lash

Abstract Having explored Sports Psychology, this chapter moves into the physical domain of actual practice. Athletes train to perform, surgeons perform to train. This has been changing over the years with technological advances facilitating the development of virtual reality simulators, an exciting move away from the rather 'dry' wet labs. This has been driven recently by a global pandemic bringing much of 'physical medicine' to a standstill. I will review the evidence for simulators in surgical training as perhaps the most obvious tool for improving 'how' surgery is done within our 'Part I' perspective. Can surgeons now train to perform at last? However, I have several questions to answer. Chapter 1 revealed the critical effects of physiological arousal and cognitive anxiety on performance but can these be replicated in a simulator? Is their usefulness limited to the very early stages of surgical training or are they useful even for experienced surgeons? The airline industry uses simulators throughout a pilot's career, surgeons use them only at the beginning. What is a learning curve *in surgery* and how might simulators influence it? Finally, might simulators actually interfere with the surgeon developing the complex schemas required to solve complex surgical problems?

Keywords Sports psychology · Surgical training · Simulation-based training · Surgeon performance · Surgical decision-making

2.1 What Has Been the Gold Standard for Training Surgeons?

Post the Enlightenment era up to the nineteenth century, surgeons learned through apprenticeships beginning around the age of 12 and lasting up to 7 years. (And I thought surgeons were looking younger these days!) The student learned through direct observation and subsequent imitation. As surgery moved from a trade to a profession the apprenticeship model continued until the end of the nineteenth century and beginning of twentieth century when training took on its modern familiar form under the influence of William Halsted (who was unfortunately also under the influence). It is summarised by the familiar quip, 'See one, do one, teach one'! Of interest this shift in training is why, in the UK, we spend years studying to gain the title 'Dr' and then the next several years trying to lose it! The surgeons were the barbers not the professionals! Halstead's principles were as follows:

- The resident must have intense and repetitive opportunities to take care of surgical patients under the supervision of a skilled surgical teacher.
- The resident must acquire an understanding of the scientific basis of surgical disease.
- The resident must acquire the skills in patient management and technical operations of increasing complexity with graded enhanced responsibility and independence.

It has been argued that 'graded enhanced responsibility' is no longer acceptable given the social and economic realities of modern-day medicine and society in general which is far less tolerant of risk. (Gill 2006; Sealy 1999). There has also been a move away from 'intense' training given the legislation reducing doctors working hours. Of interest, Halstead worked exceptionally long hours, likely fuelled by an accidental cocaine addiction, and he expected his trainees to work equally hard. Might simulators replace Halstead?

2.2 How Might Simulators Improve on Current Methods?

There are many issues with the Halsteadian approach to training including inconsistency in the levels of knowledge and skills acquired due to variations in clinical exposure, educational opportunities and, let's face it, the enthusiasm of the trainee and trainer. 'Excellent' clinical exposure to many cases does not necessarily result in an 'excellent' level of skill acquired, it does not guarantee quality or competency. Reductions in training hours due to regulations, such as the European Working Time Directive, further limit potential training opportunities as do the ethical concerns over the use of patients for training purposes and a general increase in risk aversion in society at large. Theatres are increasingly seen as too valuable a resource to be used for trainees to acquire basic surgical skills (Sachdeva et al. 2007). As a result the use of inanimate skills training stations, cadaveric and plastic models and subsequently simulators have been used to break down the surgery into smaller component parts each of which can be practised. Dexterity can be improved as can knowledge of the procedures, without exposing a patient to risk and there is an increasing body of data demonstrating excellent transference of the skills to the theatre (Sachdeva 2007).

COVID brought new challenges to all aspects of medical care and helped to push new ways of doing things. The impact on training was significant. One study, across 32 countries, described the impact as 'severe' with over 76% of trainees reporting a decrease in surgical activity of > 75% (Ferrara et al. 2020). Among other recommendations for future training there was strong agreement (nearly 90%) recommending the increased use of surgical simulators in surgical training with only around half of trainees having access currently (Ferrara et al. 2020). Given the challenges and limitations discussed, simulators seem a sensible move forward and are used in other industries with great success, notably the airline industry.

2.3 Aircraft Simulators—A Pilot's Experience

To explore this area, I interviewed a Captain of a well-known international airline who I will refer to as 'The Captain'. To understand the utility of simulators in the airline industry we need to go back through the training of a commercial pilot. As is often the case, The Captain started his flying career as a fighter pilot flying Jaguars before moving to the commercial airline industry. I imagine this must be something like retiring from Formula 1 to drive a milk cart although, as I learned, there is still plenty of drama to be had (or rather avoided!). However, in general the aspiring pilot will need to learn to fly a single-engine aircraft first and gain a private pilot licence and then move on to twin-engine planes in order to deal with the sudden loss of an engine and the resultant instability as the plane yaws. This is apparently very bad. Having attained their commercial pilot licence, they can then apply to the airlines for a job as first officer or they may be one of the few who have secured sponsorship with an airline with training naturally leading to a job, competence permitting. It is at this stage that access to a simulator is first required; the actual 'learning to fly' was real life. The job offer will be for a specific aircraft and the pilot will train on the simulator for that aircraft. Having successfully completed the simulator training and assessment the pilot is licenced to fly that aircraft. Having thought about it this makes perfect sense. I have never seen 'L' plates on a tail fin, nor would I want to board a plane with them on display! (Although much surgery is carried under exactly such an arrangement!) At a later date the pilot might get the opportunity to move from short haul to long haul or transfer airlines at which point they will need to access the specific simulator to learn to fly their next aircraft and so on. The Captain had previously flown Boeings and when he changed airlines he needed to learn the Airbus and so it was back to the simulator.

The next use of the simulator is a twice-yearly assessment of active pilots. In these sessions the pilots are not performing routine flights, they are being faced with various scenarios and emergencies. I asked The Captain about 'psychological buy in' as it is my contention that the surgeons are not performing in a realistic environment with current simulators. It does not feel real sitting in a room with a plastic model and when I have used them there is a sense of invincibility because nothing really matters, no one gets harmed there are no consequences there is no fear to control. The Captain stated that although there is an initial awareness that he is in a simulator, the flight deck is so real that when the scenarios begin, he is totally immersed and loses awareness of the simulator. It all feels very real and he will unpack his experiences well after the event. Simulators are used to expose pilots to solving various emergency situations and test and refine communication skills, situational awareness, threat and error management and the effective use of decision-making tools like 'Time, Diagnose, Options, Decide, Assign tasks, Review' (TDODAR). This is in stark contrast to surgery where the simulator is used most heavily during the initial learning period before even getting into theatre and seldom used thereafter, at least on reviewing the register of users in my unit. They are also used in isolation with no supervision or feedback other than that generated by the simulator if it is capable of providing such information.

The aviation simulator is also used to assess the team not just the pilot. The team consists of the Captain and the First Officer. There is a unique relationship between the Captain and the First Officer and their interaction is critical to the success of the flight. The Captain talked about the 'routine' when the Captain meets the First Officer for the first time before a flight and the conversation that ensues in order to gain a mutual understanding and set expectations for the flight. It is important for the Captain to know if the First Officer has just finished a long run of flights away from home as well as ensuring the First Officer knows to pull him up if he sees anything 'unusual' occurring. The Captain told me that 'unusual' usually means drifting away from a 'Standard Operating Procedure' (SOP), of which there are many, and he wants to know if he strays from these. This open and honest dialogue has much to do with the introduction of the Crew Resource Management (CRM) system that has successfully flattened the hierarchy in the cockpit.

The team in surgery is far more extensive and the relationships are very different. In surgery assistants are usually junior doctors or medical students who are learning. Being 'scrubbed in' helps them get close to the action and as involved in the case as the consultant allows. In general, a consultant's reaction to being abruptly corrected by a trainee would likely be less than pleasant. One of my very first fellows insisted on telling me how his former London consultant did absolutely everything and anything I did was immediately followed by… 'Oh, Mr Laidlaw does it like this!' Although this was a little frustrating and an assault on my fragile but developing ego, it did give me food for thought at times. Perhaps more similar to the First Officer/Captain relationship would be when two consultants are jointly working on a case and in this situation the interactions are likely to be far more open and equal. Other key relationships in theatre include the anaesthetist, in terms of keeping the patient safe, and the scrub nurse, in terms of making progress surgically, and these relationships differ in terms of significance per speciality. My anaesthetist can relax most of the time as I perform eye surgery but is all hands-on deck with big spinal procedures where control of blood pressure from bleeding is critical. It is not common to have *any* let alone *all* these people present during simulator training. Surgical development seems to be a lone venture.

2.4 Aviation and Surgery—A Literature Review

There is agreement in the literature supporting my initial observations and also the understanding I gained from my interview with The Captain. The comparisons between aviation and medicine are indeed frequent with additional comparisons in terms of use of simulators (Wood et al. 2022a, b).

Wood's paper looked specifically at the comparison of cataract surgery with short-haul flights. Similarities were identified in terms of multiple daily repetitive events within a pre-planned routine, standardised preparation, and controlled trajectory, all executed by highly trained individuals and teams in a technologically advanced environment. Both are exposed to external unpredictable events as a result of failings of humans or errors in the highly complex technical equipment (Wood et al. 2022a, b). They also highlight the importance of non-technical skills (NTS) and human factors (HF) as a more common cause of failure, in both surgery and aviation, than purely failure of technical skills (TS) (Wood et al. 2022a, b).

Wood compares how the disciplines differ in their use of simulators with experienced pilots required to undergo simulator assessment six monthly for their entire careers with no such requirements for surgeons. In another paper by Wood, it is noted that the flight-simulator physically moves around and replicates the flight deck and pilot views in immense detail, they are *immersive* (Wood et al. 2022a, b). Specific scenarios can be simulated like engine failure and even smoke in the cockpit, they feel real. This is certainly supported by my interview with The Captain. However, it is noted that current surgical simulators are typically placed in non-surgical environments and use a synthetic model with a solitary surgeon engaged. Few are truly immersive, focus on NTS or simulate specific scenarios (Lee et al. 2020; Wood et al. 2022a, b). Other differences are noted in terms of the monitoring of each activity with aircraft systems constantly monitoring performance of the plane and giving direction to the pilot when failure is detected whereas the surgeon has to monitor both the performance of the equipment and the response of the patient (Wood et al. 2022a, b). Two planes that are the same will tend to behave the same whereas no two patients will show this level of consistency and it is therefore harder to simulate failure in patients compared to aircraft.

The lack of realism, the lack of an 'immersive environment', eliminates many of the stress factors discussed in the Sports Psychology chapter and restricts full buy in, or 'adrenaline rush', by the surgeon. This is not case with aircraft simulators as attested by The Captain in our interview. Although some surgical simulators have a degree of haptic feedback, tissues do not respond as they do in real life, unlike the aircraft simulator. One of my current fellows even suggested that now he has become proficient in a specific task in real life, he would score lower on the equivalent simulated task compared to his initial scores. Aviation simulators develop and test decision-making processes in emergency situations, surgical simulators develop manual dexterity, hand eye coordination and allow rehearsal of steps in surgery. The surgical simulator is very much a 'Part I' tool, the aircraft simulator is actually much more of a 'Part III' tool. So, what is the utility of the surgical simulator? Do they shorten the learning curve of surgeons or perhaps allow them to ascend it without consequences to patients? Actually, what is a learning curve exactly?

2.5 Learning Curves—An Exploration

We all talk about them, but what do we actually know about them? What is a learning curve? A learning curve is a graphical representation of how proficient people are at a task and the amount of experience they have in performing that task. Proficiency is measured on the Y-axis and experience on the X-axis. The curve has nothing to do with the difficulty of a specific task; it indicates the rate of change in performing a task with increasing proficiency over time. A 'steep learning curve' is often used to indicate a 'difficult to learn' task; however the curve actually shows rapid progress in a very short time, a 'very easy to learn' task! Learning curves come in different shapes; straight line, exponential, exponential with a limit and sigmoid to name a few common shapes (See Fig. 2.1).

The history of learning curves quickly moved from psychology to manufacturing. Herman Ebbinghaus first described a 'shaped curve' following subjects' performance in memorising random syllables in 1885 in the field of psychology and learning and showed the 'curves' could go up and down and even oscillate (Ebbinghaus 1913). The first actual mention of a 'learning curve' was in 1899 from studies on the acquisition of telegraphic language (Bryan and Harter 1899). The concept was applied to manufacturing aeroplanes in 1936 and was known as the 'experience curve' (Wright 1936). Learning curves entered medicine in the early 1980s and have been applied variously to many aspects of healthcare but with little rigour in terms of design and analysis (Ramsay et al. 2000). The learning curve was also blamed for high

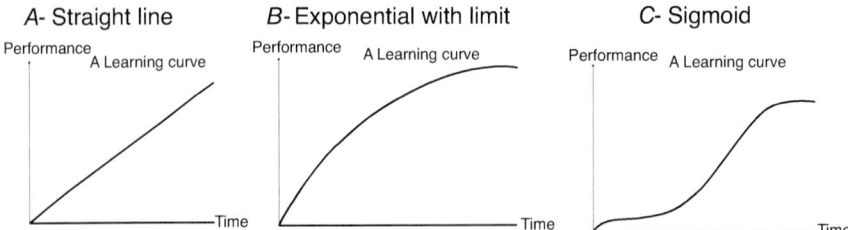

Fig. 2.1 Examples of learning curves

death rates in children undergoing Heart surgery in Bristol in the late 1990s (Ramsay 1999). I remember this particular incident well as I was a medical student on a surgical placement at the time and the consultant, a very senior, 'old school' (looked like a WW1 fighter pilot complete with moustache but lacking the outstretched white scarf and yet also incredibly personable), asked us the question, 'How long is a learning curve?' I am still not sure we have answered this question. The term has permeated surgical training and practice but how useful is it as a concept let alone a practical benchmark?

2.6   A Surgical Learning Curve?

None of the curves in Fig. 2.1 resonate with my experience in surgery, they are too simple. Learning curves actually function on multiple levels. Progress on these curves can be viewed at the macro-level, making progress in surgical procedures (hip replacement, cataract surgery, etc.) or on the micro-level, making progress through specific individual manoeuvres which then build together to form the macro-level procedure. The micro-level consists of dozens of micro-manoeuvres *each* with its own learning curve. There is also an initial learning curve as the trainee gets used to the tools of the trade, not just holding and using instruments but also using microscopes in the case of ophthalmology, ENT, neurosurgery, etc., or laparoscopic viewing systems. There is not only the micro to macro-level of the learning curves but also the environment in which the learning occurs. Models and simulators are the most controlled and predictable environments and facilitate isolation of individual learning curves in a manufacturing-type manner. The Eyesi ophthalmic simulator is able to measure time and movement accurately which is ideal for the micro-level learning typical early on in training. In theatre, strict case selection and supervision can only replicate a degree of this control and predictability and psychological and physiological effects start to influence the learning curve. Control and predictability reduce with a less selective and more complex case mix resulting in new applications of existing learning curves, flattening of the curves and even reversal of the curve at times in more difficult cases. Finally, dealing with complications represents further loss of control and predictability, even more so when the trainee is operating alone, further influencing the learning curve. Running a theatre on your own requires a learning curve!

On both the micro and the macro-level the curve flattens, the law of diminishing returns and eventually plateaus, as techniques learned imbed and become more predictable and streamlined. Even at the plateau stage I believe there is variability with some surgeons keen to continue to stretch and push outside their comfort zone and innovate and extend the boundaries of surgery, whilst others are content to remain comfortable (although this very much strays into 'Part III'). However, at some point the curve starts to decline either through overconfidence, taking on a more challenging case mix or, for us all eventually, cognitive and physical decline. Retirement age varies in different countries from the age of 60 in Russia and China to (currently) 68 in the UK. But with ongoing pension reforms and declining birth rates threatening to push the retirement age out further, one must perhaps consider how high the curve got and how quickly it falls to an 'unsafe' height before making judgments on how safe a surgeon is to continue. Ideally, they will have the insight to 'quit whilst they are ahead'.

With time the surgeon builds up a 'toolbox' that can be used on subsequent learning curves as new methods and technologies arise. I explain this to my fellows using the analogy of Tarzan swinging from vine to vine. They must be careful the gap between vines is not too wide for them; however, there will be inevitable 'stretch' and even 'air'. Surgeons will need to embrace new learning curves throughout their careers as technology advances and this can be stressful, especially as it seems that 'Neuroticism' increases with age. (more 'Part III' territory) I remember feeling that I had transitioned from 'technician' to 'surgeon' only when I started to manage my own complications and as a consultant, I have embarked on several learning curves over my career thus far.

Figure 2.2 represents my personal learning curve for a new technique that I learned as a consultant, i.e. without 'supervision'. I learned by reading papers, watching videos, endless visualisation/imagery, strict prospective audit and, of great importance and benefit, chatting the technique through with a couple of trusted colleagues sharing our experiences as we learned together. I did not have access to an appropriate simulator and did not use model eyes but extended techniques I was already using. The model eyes failed to replicate the tissue responses. My first case was probably the best case in my first 50 and took less than thirty minutes to complete much to the admiration of a group of Fellows who had come along especially to watch the new technique! They were most impressed. The second case, completed immediately after the first but thankfully after the impressed fellows had left, was abandoned after two hours! You will note that I have assumed 'time' to be the metric underlying performance here. There were certainly times I questioned continuing and the 'more complex case dip' was repeated many times. It even became apparent the technique had a different complication profile depending on which eye I was operating on. I am still discovering complications at over 300 cases but they are rare now. Surgical time has reduced both in terms of duration and variability which indicates increased efficiency and accuracy of movements. I do not operate 'faster' just more efficiently getting each step *Right First Time*'. ('Part II' territory). It could be I am a slow learner or it could be that we all underestimate the actual time it takes to climb whatever learning curve we are on to reach a 'safe height' or even the 'peak' height on the plateau. I think we are in danger of accepting a competence level way below what it could be with significantly more experience in our own hands or accepting a height way below someone else's?

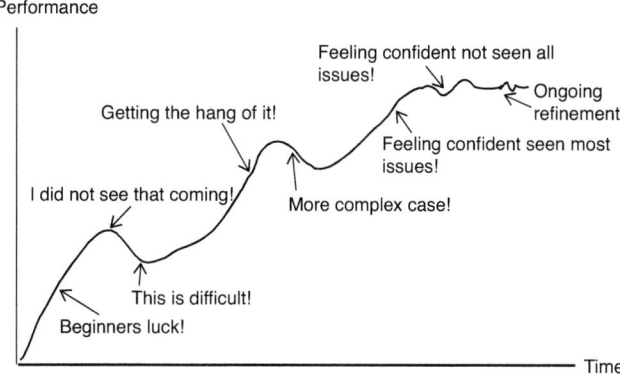

Fig. 2.2 My most recent learning curve experience—Scleral Haptic Fixation

2.7 Theoretical and Practical Issues

Having explored the history, concepts and experience of learning curves what is the actual evidence for their usefulness? Unfortunately, analysing learning curves has historically been insufficient to influence practice (Valsamis et al. 2018). This is perhaps, not surprising given the complexities discussed. Do we assess on the macro (procedural)-level or the micro (individual steps)-level? If we limit analysis to the micro-level, we can lose sight at the macro-level but then the macro-level performance is a direct consequence of micro-level proficiency. What should be on the 'performance' Y-axis? Intuitively the time taken to complete a task should reduce as one gets better and time is very easy to measure. This underlies Taylorism (scientific management theory) and production line experience curves. However, is faster better? Should 'quality of technique' be on the Y-axis but if so, how do we measure this? Is it accuracy of movements or number of movements to accomplish a task? This may end up including accurate but unnecessary movements? If we want to move away from a simple qualitative analysis, how do we analyse results mathematically and how do we then compare surgeons or benchmark?

When is a learning curve 'complete', at what 'height' do we assess competence and what determines this threshold, time, quality or both? Is it only finally reached on the plateau phase? From Fig. 2.2, I appear to have reached a short plateau phase twice before the final plateau and at significantly lower heights than the final summit. Might we accept lower standards of excellence due to an impatience to arrive? With any technical task some people will simply perform much better than others and so achieve a greater plateau height. The elite athletes in sport and the Virtuosos in music demonstrate the actual heights that can be attained, way in excess of the average or even the excellent performer. Are we really happy with plus or minus 2 standard deviations (95% of all surgeons within) or even plus or minus 1 standard deviation

(66% of all surgeons within) as a measure of acceptable competence as per current audit requirements? Where is excellence? Do we simply want to be 'safe'? Can you imagine the response of patients to all this and what about the surgeons who assume (as all seem to) that they are above average?

If I zoom out of all these details and reflect on trainees in the real world, I see two useful time aspects to the learning curve and one physical observation worth exploring. A junior trainee performing an 'easy' case takes a certain amount of time and a 'difficult' case much more time. However, as they become more experienced the *time* taken to complete the surgery reduces as does the *variability* in time between cases including the more difficult cases. This was also my personal experience as detailed above. Time taken is a very good surrogate for quality but not completely. Fast surgery might simply be the result of the surgeon rushing and preforming suboptimally. Movement represents a good 'physical' aspect to progress up the learning curve. The expert's 'intention to execution ratio' will be close to 1:1 whereas the novice may take several attempts to complete each manoeuvre. Ideally, the overall technique becomes increasingly streamlined, eliminating unnecessary manoeuvres and tends towards 'Lean' which I will explore in 'Part II'. Evidence for time, accuracy and variability is explored in a study by Mahr and Hodge with 12 residents and 3 experienced surgeons performing anti-tremor training on the Eyesi simulator (Ophthalmology). It is at the micro-level but did demonstrate that experienced surgeons had 76% more precise surgical outcomes and more consistent scores in time and accuracy (Mahr and Hodge 2008). It is a very small study and it would be interesting to compare 12 experienced surgeons in pursuit of excellence.

Learning curves are complex and analysis of them has failed to be of any significant clinical benefit. However, in exploring aspects of time and motion, especially at the micro-level, there might be substrate for exploring their utility in the realm of the simulator. I still have significant questions over the height however!

2.8 Simulators in Surgery—The Evidence

In terms of the evidence for the effectiveness and validity of simulator training in improving skills, robust frameworks such as Messicks Validity Framework are generally absent (93% in one review study) in favour of the more subjective 'face validity' (Borgersen et al. 2018; Lee et al. 2020). This is important given that validity is critical in evaluating the claims made by these studies. The validity of simulators as representing the 'real world' needs inputs from experts in the field rather than subjective impressions from novice participants, often medical students. Lee found a quarter of studies used medical students, not practising surgeons, further limiting applicability to the real world (Lee et al. 2020).

The structure and assessment of standards for technical performance of simulator training is also lacking with one review finding only 37 studies out of over 1800 setting such standards (Goldenberg et al. 2016). There is a lack of educational theoretical foundations such as 'Kolbs Experiential Learning theory' where concrete learning experiences, reflective observation, abstract conceptualisation and active experimentation are used to guide trainees through their learning experience (Poore et al. 2014).

Appropriate validity and educational frameworks are sadly lacking in many studies restricting their usefulness; however, it would be useful to know if they benefit patients and healthcare systems by reducing complications in the real world and perhaps shortening the training period. These questions reside at the start of the learning curve but are they also able to differentiate between novice and expert surgeons suggesting utility further up the curve?

2.9 Simulator Evidence—Effect on the Learning Curve—*Length*

As discussed, to be effective, simulator training needs to be validated as representing the real world, structured within a standardised curriculum including knowledge-based learning, along a step-wise technical skills pathway, with ongoing feedback rather than simply improving specific technical skills (Feudner et al. 2009; Spiteri et al. 2014). We will explore these concepts reviewing studies using the Eyesi Surgical simulator which has the strongest validity evidence of any ophthalmic simulator currently (Lee et al. 2020).

Like any surgery, cataract surgery is comprised of multiple (micro-level) technical procedural steps which must all be mastered. Failure in any step can lead to a complication or a surgical path that subsequently veers 'off Piste'. An important and challenging step to learn is the capsulorrhexis where a round opening is made in the capsule of the lens giving access to the cataract and providing an opening through which to place the new plastic lens. This step is carried out very early in the surgery and so suboptimal performance here can result in further complications during and after surgery. Being able to practice this step with a simulator could be of benefit in the real world both in terms of time taken to complete it and accuracy in terms of size and shape and the number and nature of manoeuvres. Fuedner found that residents and medical students trained on the Eyesi simulator performed better compared to non-training controls in subsequent wet lab assessment, so *not* real world (Feudner et al. 2009). Daly found Simulators were comparable to training in a wet lab among ophthalmology residents (Daly et al. 2013; Feudner et al. 2009). Both were small studies which do limit findings and also involved medical students. Perhaps these simply demonstrate that practice, whether on a simulator or in a wet lab, will improve performance at a very specific motor task? However, the Eyesi simulator uses training modules which measure five specific aspects of surgery; target achievement, efficiency, instrument utilisation, tissue damage and microscope usage. This analysis provides much richer feedback to the trainee as compared to a wet lab and enables us to populate the Y-axis with both time and motion over experience on the X-axis. There is evidence that the learning curve can be shortened with virtual reality simulator training compared to traditional cadaveric training in laparoscopic cholecystectomy surgery also suggesting more is going on than simply practice (Aggarwal et al. 2007). This would support the concept of shortening the learning curve.

Studies on construct validity (the extent to which the test or measure accurately assesses what it's supposed to) have shown that the Eyesi can distinguish between novice and intermediate *or* experienced surgeons but not between intermediate *and* experienced surgeons (Mahr and Hodge 2008; Spiteri et al. 2014). Spiteri looked at novices (<10 cases), intermediate (50–200 cases) and experienced (>500 cases) cataract surgeons with construct validity defined as the ability to differentiate these three groups based on simulator-derived metrics covering nine tasks (four abstract— grasping shapes, etc., and five procedural—three on capsulorrhexis and two on phacoemulsification). The intermediate and experienced group showed no differences on all the abstract tasks and some of the procedural tasks indicating a plateau phase of the learning curve suggesting that inexperienced learners will benefit most from this type of curriculum training (Spiteri et al. 2014). This would suggest an effect on shortening the learning curve only up to a certain height but above that, no significant effect. This suggests they are most useful at the beginning of the learning curve only.

2.10 Simulator Evidence—Effect on the Learning Curve—*Height*

If we define a certain 'height' as the threshold of competence required in order to progress to actual patients there is good evidence, early on in the learning curve, that simulator experience does transfer to a real-world reduction in complications (Lee et al. 2020). A UK multicentre retrospective study involving 265 ophthalmology trainees in their first two years showed that complication rates dropped from 4.2 to 2.6% (38% reduction) following the introduction of Eyesi simulators into training programmes (Ferris et al. 2020). In another study, it was demonstrated that participating in simulation-based training prior to undertaking cataract surgery for the first time was associated with significantly reduced risks of posterior capsular rupture and vitreous prolapse (Staropoli et al. 2018).

It does seem that, in spite of the poor methodology and issues over construct validity and educational frameworks, the use of simulators does result in a reduction in real-world complications for early trainees. However, this effect seems to be limited to the start of the learning curve.

2.11 Simulators and Real-Life Surgery—An Analogy to Reading

Imagine learning to read where the letters are constantly presented in different fonts? Surgical manoeuvres on patients can feel very different from patient to patient. The simulator provides this initial consistency and predictability to get the trainee started. They can learn how to hold and use instruments. Once recognition of letters has been achieved the next stage is the sound the letters make. The instruments can be used in the simulator with predictable and consistent results. The effects of this tissue manipulation can be monitored and measured providing rich feedback and further refinement of skill. Next, sounds have to be blended to make words and words can be put together into sentences. Similarly, sequences of surgical manoeuvres are put together to form the basics of technique and simulators are well positioned to deliver this as sequences of movements that can be practised, assessed and then refined in terms of time and movement. Then reading can move to the meaning within the sentences, with less effort now required by the reader as they no longer see individual letters, they just read words. Surgically less effort is required on the actual mechanical movements and more attention can be given to putting them together in sequences. Simulators can still deliver this although I think we are reaching their useful limit. We will explore System 1 and 2 later in 'Part III', but suffice it to say that simulators allow the storage of basic technique allowing it to become automatic. Next sentences have meaning in the context of paragraphs and we begin to understand that a story is being told although we do not know what the story is. The story is beyond the words and sentences but includes them. In the same way surgery starts to become about the interaction of the technique with the tissues and their responses which can be variable and all this must occur within a plan to solve a problem. This is where I believe simulators, at the current level of development, cease to be of benefit. Decision making plays an increasingly important role as appropriate techniques need to be selected, variability is introduced, predictability of tissue response reduces and control reduces. Surgery begins to move out of 'Part I' and into 'Parts II and III'. In the real world, psychology begins to factor in and responses to stress have an effect as we discussed in Chap. 1. Simulators cannot model this currently. Finally, surgery introduces curve balls with complications. The surgeon must use extensive knowledge and experience to navigate these to arrive at the intended destination. We are now firmly into 'Part III', and it is here that simulators may have a detrimental effect on progression. Yu et al. criticised the literature on simulators suggesting that physiological and psychological perspectives were not taken into account (Yu et al. 2022). They drew upon the work of Sweller and cognitive load theory and schema theory to suggest that simulators might actually encourage deficient problem-solving techniques, in terms of the total surgical pathway, preventing the formation of schemas known to be used by expert problems solvers (Sweller 1988). We will cover this in more detail in 'Part III'.

2.12   Conclusion

If our perspective remains firmly in 'Part I' simulators have a lot to offer at the beginning of the learning curve, specifically, at the micro-level and basic procedural level. Analysis of learning curves is somewhat complex with no useful quantitative analysis studies that might influence practice to date however, in exploring these difficulties two properties emerge as important to consider, 'time' and 'poverty of movement'. The 'Eyesi' simulator can measure both time and movement in multiple dimensions and can give feedback to the surgeon facilitating progression through marginal gains in each aspect. This results in a shortening of the learning curve allowing a certain 'height' to be reached more quickly. Practically this results in a reduction in real-world complications, saving healthcare costs, patient distress and theatre time. In a competitive and resource limited Halstedian world, simulators provide opportunities for regular practice. Surgeons can train to perform rather than perform to train. However, simulators are currently less useful to the experienced surgeon with the Eyesi simulator unable to differentiate between intermediate and experienced surgeons. However, surgery at this more advanced level seems to move out of 'Part I' into 'Part II' and even more so into 'Part III' where decision making and problem solving become paramount and it is at this level that simulators might actually interfere with learning. It may be with time, AI could introduce variability and complexity within a truly immersive virtual reality environment including all team members allowing more psychological buy in, developing NTS and even modelling complications, but not yet.

2.13   To Try

Try drawing a learning curve for a common procedure you perform.

What aspects of the surgery are you considering when drawing the curve?

What metric did you apply to the 'Y'-axis (performance)?

What features, both internal to the surgeon and external did you draw upon to influence the shape of the curve?

Did it fit with the classic shapes in the figures above?

If you have access to a simulator, do you actually use it?

How can you get the most out of your sessions? Do you have scoring matrices, learning objectives, educational frameworks, mentors or supervisors?

Do you audit your results?

If you do not use it, why not? This is a good indication of how useful you *really* think they are!

Do you agree with my conclusions on their limitations as your experience increases?

Do they help you in managing complications?

References

Aggarwal R, Ward J, Balasundaram I, Sains P, Athanasiou T, Darzi A. Proving the effectiveness of virtual reality simulation for training in laparoscopic surgery. Ann Surg. 2007;246(5):771–9. https://doi.org/10.1097/SLA.0b013e3180f61b09.

Borgersen NJ, Naur TMH, Sørensen SMD, Bjerrum F, Konge L, Subhi Y, Thomsen ASS. Gathering validity evidence for surgical simulation. Ann Surg. 2018;267(6):1063–8. https://doi.org/10.1097/SLA.0000000000002652.

Bryan WL, Harter N. Studies on the telegraphic language: the acquisition of a hierarchy of habits. Psychol Rev. 1899;6(4):345–75. https://doi.org/10.1037/h0073117.

Daly MK, Gonzalez E, Siracuse-Lee D, Legutko PA. Efficacy of surgical simulator training versus traditional wet-lab training on operating room performance of ophthalmology residents during the capsulorhexis in cataract surgery. J Cataract Refract Surg. 2013;39(11):1734–41. https://doi.org/10.1016/j.jcrs.2013.05.044.

Ebbinghaus H. Memory: a contribution to experimental psychology. Teachers College Press. 1913. https://doi.org/10.1037/10011-000.

Ferrara M, Romano V, Steel DH, Gupta R, Iovino C, van Dijk EHC, Ferrara M, Romano V, Steel DH, Gupta R, Iovino C, van Dijk EHC, Rocha-de-Lossada C, Bali E, Valldeperas X, Romano D, Gadhvi KA, Matarazzo F, Tzamalis A, Romano MR (2020). Reshaping ophthalmology training after COVID-19 pandemic. Eye 34(11):2089–97. https://doi.org/10.1038/s41433-020-1061-3

Ferris, J. D., Donachie, P. H., Johnston, R. L., Barnes, B., Olaitan, M., & Sparrow, J. M. (2020). Royal College of Ophthalmologists' National Ophthalmology Database study of cataract surgery: report 6. The impact of EyeSi virtual reality training on complications rates of cataract surgery performed by first and second year trainees. *British Journal of Ophthalmology*, *104*(3), 324–9. https://doi.org/10.1136/bjophthalmol-2018-313817

Feudner EM, Engel C, Neuhann IM, Petermeier K, Bartz-Schmidt K-U, Szurman P. Virtual reality training improves wet-lab performance of capsulorhexis: results of a randomized, controlled study. Graefe's Arch Clin Exp Ophthal. 2009;247(7):955–63. https://doi.org/10.1007/s00417-008-1029-7.

Gill T. No Fear. Calouste Gulbenkian Foundation: Growing up in a risk averse Society; 2006.

Goldenberg MG, Garbens A, Szasz P, Hauer T, Grantcharov TP. Systematic review to establish absolute standards for technical performance in surgery. Br J Surg. 2016;104(1):13–21. https://doi.org/10.1002/bjs.10313.

Lee R, Raison N, Lau WY, Aydin A, Dasgupta P, Ahmed K, Haldar S. A systematic review of simulation-based training tools for technical and non-technical skills in ophthalmology. Eye. 2020;34(10):1737–59. https://doi.org/10.1038/s41433-020-0832-1.

Mahr MA, Hodge DO. Construct validity of anterior segment anti-tremor and forceps surgical simulator training modules. J Cataract Refract Surg. 2008;34(6):980–5. https://doi.org/10.1016/j.jcrs.2008.02.015.

Poore JA, Cullen DL, Schaar GL. Simulation-based interprofessional education guided by Kolb's experiential learning theory. Clin Simul Nurs. 2014;10(5):e241–7. https://doi.org/10.1016/j.ecns.2014.01.004.

Ramsay CR, Grant AM, Wallace SA, Garthwaite PH, Monk AF, Russell IT. Assessment of the learning curve in health technologies a systematic review. Int J Technol Assess Health Care. 2000;16(04):S0266462300103149. https://doi.org/10.1017/S0266462300103149.

Ramsay S. Bristol surgeon attributes poor performance to "learning curve." The Lancet. 1999;354(9194):1980. https://doi.org/10.1016/S0140-6736(05)76752-0.

Sachdeva AK. The changing paradigm of residency education in surgery: a perspective from the American college of surgeons. Am Surg. 2007;73(2):120–9. https://doi.org/10.1177/000313480707300206.

Sachdeva AK, Bell RH, Britt LD, Tarpley JL, Blair PG, Tarpley MJ. National efforts to reform residency education in surgery. Acad Med. 2007;82(12):1200–10. https://doi.org/10.1097/ACM.0b013e318159e052.

Sealy WC. Halsted is dead: time for change in graduate surgical education. Curr Surg. 1999;56(1–2):34–9. https://doi.org/10.1016/S0149-7944(99)00005-7.

Spiteri AV, Aggarwal R, Kersey TL, Sira M, Benjamin L, Darzi AW, Bloom PA. Development of a virtual reality training curriculum for phacoemulsification surgery. Eye. 2014;28(1):78–84. https://doi.org/10.1038/eye.2013.211.

Staropoli PC, Gregori NZ, Junk AK, Galor A, Goldhardt R, Goldhagen BE, Shi W, Feuer W. Surgical simulation training reduces intraoperative cataract surgery complications among residents. Simulat Healthcare: J Soc Simul Healthcare. 2018;13(1):11–5. https://doi.org/10.1097/SIH.0000000000000255.

Sweller J. Cognitive load during problem solving: effects on learning. Cogn Sci. 1988;12(2):257–85. https://doi.org/10.1207/s15516709cog1202_4.

Valsamis EM, Chouari T, O'Dowd-Booth C, Rogers B, Ricketts D. Learning curves in surgery: variables, analysis and applications. Postgrad Med J. 2018;94(1115):525–30. https://doi.org/10.1136/postgradmedj-2018-135880.

Wood TC, Maqsood S, Sancha W, Nanavaty MA, Rajak S. Comparisons between cataract surgery and aviation. Eye. 2022a;36(3):490–1. https://doi.org/10.1038/s41433-021-01877-4.

Wood TC, Maqsood S, Sancha W, Saunders A, Lockington D, Nanavaty MA, Rajak S. Principles of simulation and their role in enhancing cataract surgery training. Eye. 2022b;36(8):1529–31. https://doi.org/10.1038/s41433-022-02052-z.

Wright TP. Factors affecting the cost of airplanes. J Aeronaut Sci. 1936;3(4):122–8. https://doi.org/10.2514/8.155.

Yu P, Pan J, Wang Z, Shen Y, Li J, Hao A, Wang H. Quantitative influence and performance analysis of virtual reality laparoscopic surgical training system. BMC Med Educ. 2022;22(1):92. https://doi.org/10.1186/s12909-022-03150-y.

Chapter 3
Performance—What Can We Learn from Musicians?

It's a shame we celebrate mediocrity and compare at adequate.
—Stephen Lash

Currently, practicing surgery is a bit like practicing your golf swing in the dark, with a blindfold in a competition with no prize!
—Stephen Lash

Abstract My chapter on elite athletes and Sports Psychology attempted to extract techniques for enhancing the surgeon's performance in the moment of, and the preparation for, surgery. I examined technique at the micro-level looking for marginal gains. However, athletes are tested regularly in competitions and ranked. Their performances are manifest and can easily be judged, less so for surgeons. Simulators help the surgeon 'practice to perform' but only at the start of the learning curve. How is performance enhanced at higher levels and how would we know if we succeeded? In this chapter I want to look at musicians and what might be learned from them in terms of performance, practice and virtuosity. I want to ask the question 'are we aiming high enough as surgeons?' Like athletes, a musician's performance is more manifest and more easily judged than a surgeons' but it does have a greater 'subjective' element. I want to investigate what it takes to become very good, to become exceptional to become a concert pianist, and then see what might be imitated in the pursuit of greatness and the level of commitment required. Can we achieve virtuosity in surgery?

Keywords Surgeon's performance · Musicians · Deliberate practice · Practice regimes · Simulators · Technical prowess · Patient outcomes · Surgical decision-making

S. Lash, *Improving Surgical Skills and Outcomes*,
https://doi.org/10.1007/978-3-031-66690-2_3

3.1   Introduction

I have reviewed several aspects of Sports Psychology with elite athletes that may be useful for enhancing the surgeon's performance *in* theatre and, to some extent, their preparation *for* theatre. However, professional athletes are ranked according to results, are constantly challenged in their rank by ongoing competition and their performances can be dissected by pundits for entertainment and coaches for refinement. Elite athletes are rare, talented, physiologically and even anatomically 'adapted' (Adam Peaty) and extremely driven. Performance quality is evident, manifest and critical to their continuing success and, with great rewards at stake, it is the perfect environment to seek perfection. Pushed by fear of failure and pulled towards the prize at the same time. This feels like a very different environment to that of surgeons whose performances are far less obvious, less manifest and very difficult to compare. As for trying to match the practice regimes of elite athletes, simulators seem to run out of steam beyond the basics and are hardly a good comparison to the athlete training for many hours every day. Insights from Sports Psychology, especially imagery, can offer a type of regular practice without the need for an operating theatre and patient; however, it is limited to techniques the surgeon has actually performed in real life, and it does not result in technical extension beyond them. The surgeon cannot imagine what they have not done.

Musicians can also offer insight in to performance and although, once again, the performance is manifest, evident, assessable by experts and comparisons between musicians can be made it is less binary than competitive sport, more subjective and therefore perhaps more applicable to surgery? Musicians certainly 'train' or rather 'practice' to perform but have the advantage over surgeons in that their instrument is accessible at all times and useful for progress even at virtuoso level. Interestingly, musicians might make better surgeons. In a study of 30 novice medical students asked to perform a task on a laparoscopic simulator, those currently playing an instrument completed the task significantly faster than those who did not play an instrument. This was thought to be due to enhanced visuospatial abilities developed by playing a musical instrument (Boyd et al. 2008). The complex interactions between various brain regions that come together to create music might also be involved in surgery. As part of writing this book I decided to pick up my electric guitar after thirty years and attempt to learn a difficult guitar solo. Having not really learned a new skill for many years this in itself provided insight in to my surgery and into training surgeons. I had to break the task down into small steps, get the notes correct and then put them together at a painfully slow pace. I had to work on micro-technique with alternate and sweep picking. I had to break through the feeling that I could not do it, that it was too difficult for me. It required stretch, including physical stretch for my hands and hardening of the skin on the tips of my fingers. But slowly, with repeated daily practice, I built each section up until it became automatic and then I could work on speed and finally put it all together. There is no way I could have achieved this level by booking several gigs, 'giving it a go' each time! I wish I could work on surgery in a similar manner.

Czudek, in his article 'What does it take to become a concert pianist?', highlighted several aspects which I will apply to the surgical arena (Czudek 2023). These include deliberate practice, talent, love for music, age, time availability and a good teacher. What does it take to become a concert pianist and what might it take to become a 'virtuoso' surgeon?

3.2   Deliberate Practice

Deliberate practice has been accepted for many years as a necessary component for acquiring expertise in any given discipline including sport and music. However, musical practice must be 'deliberate rather than just "playing around", and include all the relevant activities required to improve performance'(Ericsson 1993). Ericsson introduced the arbitrary '10,000-hour rule' made popular, and perhaps given more specificity than intended, by Gladwell in his book 'Outliers: The Story of Success' (Gladwell 2009). 'Hard work beats talent when talent fails to work hard' as Kevin Durant the Basketball player once quoted. However, more recent studies have built on Ericsson's work suggesting that practice alone is not sufficient to reach the heights of a virtuoso and other factors come into play including general intelligence and domain-specific intelligence or musical intelligence, which includes technical and expressive abilities (Ruthsatz et al. 2008).

Most musicians own their own instruments; few, if any, surgeons own their own simulator! A surgical simulator's benefit is most likely limited to the early part of the learning curve with the most validated ophthalmic simulator currently unable to differentiate intermediate and expert surgeons (Spiteri et al. 2014). A musical instrument has no such limitations, the learning continues uninhibited by stage from novice to virtuoso. In reality surgeons practice in a theatre, they perform to practice. It is impossible to imagine a musician adopting this strategy. High-volume super-specialist surgeons like Akahoshi Takayuki do become very good in terms of their results in comparison to 'gold audit standards' (more on this later as I question the 'Carat' of this gold), low complication rates (by yet more 'gold standards') and high levels of efficiency in terms of the numbers of cases on a list which also has much to do with the organisation of theatre not just the technical prowess of the surgeon. The push towards high volumes may underly the increasing 'super-specialisation' seen in surgery. Surgeon experience, rather than practice, seems the best correlate for musicians practice although I am sure Ericsson would describe this as 'playing around' rather than deliberate practice. Surgeons have yet to find a way to practice like musicians and I have to wonder what surgery might look like years after the day this is possible given the awe-inspiring performances of some musicians and even, if I may say so, my modest progress on that guitar solo. However, considering that playing a musical instrument involves a higher level of complex fine movements compared to the more standardised movemenets in surgery, there may not be enough complexity in surgical techniques to allow for the same kind of virtuosity to develop. Perhaps musical virtuosity predominantly resides in 'Part I' and is very visible whereas in surgery, virtuosity resides in the other, less visible boxes? I will explore this later.

3.3 Talent

Practice is essential but studies have shown that practice alone is not sufficient to become a virtuoso, talent is required. Studies have confirmed this in relation to possible hours practised by looking at the performance of children in music competitions. They found that that differing potential practice hours did not account for the rankings at this early stage, some children just won more competitions than others, they were more 'talented' (Ruthsatz et al. 2008). Talent might simply accelerate progress up the learning curve and to be truly great extensive practice is required. Ericsson found that the most talented violinists practised the most hours (Ericsson 1993). Having trained many surgeons, I can retrospectively recognise aspects of performance that I had previously thought of as talent. Talent as an accelerator is an interesting hypothesis and I certainly tend to rate speed of acquisition of skills as a strong indicator of talent. However, some people are able to learn more quickly and so appear talented but then plateau early. I have also trained slower learners whose learning curves seem to be shallow in comparison, but with a continuous incline. Learning is embedded and a higher plateau is ultimately reached. Is talent the incline, the height or perhaps both in terms of the learning curve?

Even beyond talent and practice, general intelligence has also been correlated with musical ability with a positive correlation found between general intelligence and three separate tests for musicality (Lynn and Gault 1986). General intelligence is certainly required to gain entrance to medical school and competition is significant in many surgical specialities further reducing the number of successful candidates. Domain-specific talent, which includes technical and expressive abilities, has also been shown to be important in achieving virtuosity (Ruthsatz et al. 2008). I am not sure what the correlate for 'domain-specific talent' is in surgery although Vouhe (a paediatric cardiac surgeon) has some interesting thoughts on this. Vouhe asserts that musical virtuosity consists of style, rhythm, rapidity and risk taking which are all elements beyond the actual musical score. He suggests this compares well with good surgery in that there is a balance between strictly adhering to the surgical steps required and improvising when issues arise (Vouhé 2011).

3.4 Love for Music

Love for music is often tested early on, when the child gets impatient and refuses to practice (perhaps more a test for the parents!) or, much later on, when the budding musician has reached a plateau or progress slows. This 'loss of love' maybe because they are not as good as they had hoped and enthusiasm wanes or other interests take precedent as the 'childlike' joy of the child gives way to the 'distractions' of adolescence. A love for music is important in order to traverse these inevitable stages and push on to mastery. Love for surgery? Senior and highly experienced surgeons I respect and value seem to 'love' what they do. I come to this conclusion from a variety of observations. They are focussed on surgery and interested in improving and learning new techniques even at later stages of their career with little to prove. They are very happy to enter into conversations about surgery at any time and tend to discuss their failures as well as their successes. Ego seems to be in check, humility present and as a result I never leave a conversation with one feeling one upped! Perhaps these observations are good surrogates for a love of surgery? Making a surgical career choice based on a passion for the speciality is to be encouraged rather than pursuit of secondary gain like lifestyle or income. I think the best surgeons are most likely purists and enthusiasts who, to quote Kierkegaard 'will one thing'. They are working away in some obscure hospital theatre somewhere to an audience of 1 (the patient). Beautiful things don't ask for attention, perhaps talented surgeons don't either?

3.5 Age

Children learn more quickly than adults because of their rapidly developing brains as a result of exuberant synaptogenesis. The earlier they learn the better. Mozart started at the age of 3. There are very few concert pianists who started in their late teens and none that started as an adult. In the nineteenth century, surgeons started training around the age of 12 and had to be technically excellent to avoid death (of the patient). Currently, most surgeons start around the age of 25. We are all late starters now and I am not proposing a return to the apprenticeship model in the barber shops of old London town!

3.6 Time Availability

It takes, on average, around 15 years to become a concert pianist. This is 15 years of 3–5 h per day of deliberate practice as well as studying under the best teachers (Czudek 2023). The struggle is guaranteed, success is not. Even once surgeons start, surgery is only one aspect of the training with clinical work, exam preparation, research, audit and administration all taking up time. There is a drive to reduce the training period with the current shortage of doctors in the UK. Finally, policies and restrictions on training exampled by the 'European Working Time Directive' further reduce exposure to surgery. We start late (age 25 not 3), finish earlier (around 7–9 years of training in the UK not 15) and gain far less experience (around 4 surgical sessions per week not daily exposure) compared to musicians. Every surgical activity needs to be squeezed for all the learning it can offer. Ultimately there is absolutely no comparison to musicians when it comes to time availability.

3.7 Teacher (Coach)

A good teacher is essential in order to learn a musical instrument, it is a very complex task. The teacher has to teach basic technique and theory but also has to be able to coach and develop the skills of the student, push them appropriately and encourage them but also correct them. The relationship between the student and teacher is very important, even critical to success especially at elite levels. In surgery it is sometimes possible to work for a specific consultant to gain specific experience but generally the surgeon works for various consultants with varying attitudes to teaching throughout training. There is no formal training for most consultants in terms of the education and training of trainees. I had consultants I learned a lot from and seemed to make good progress with and others less so. I am sure some of my trainees make good progress with me but others less so, it is a two-way relationship. Eventually the trainee builds up a toolbox of various techniques and approaches drawn from many consultants. What they feel is best 'in their hands'. In this way surgical teaching tends to be more like imitation with a defined end point (Consultant post), whereas in sport and music, the teacher is alongside the performer regardless of how experienced they are and training is less about imitation and more about observation and direction and is perhaps even more critical at elite levels. In fact, the coach is usually less 'able' at the elite level than the performer. This is very obvious in sport. I am sure Usain Bolt's coach would not beat him at the 100 m but clearly offered valuable advice. Training works reasonably well for trainees but as consultants it becomes very difficult. Consultants tend to work alone, there are significant pressures to deliver care and, I will argue in 'Part II', the culture is not conducive to failure. These factors make coaching difficult. Introducing 'surgical coaches' into surgery would require a complete shift in mindset for consultant surgeons, a shift away from the assumption of imitation towards a greater appreciation for knowledge and observation in the pursuit of excellence. Criticism must become subordinate to the pursuit of excellence and far less personal. Interestingly, in Clive Woodward's book 'Winning' he remarked that the most talented players were the one most keen to learn from the coaches (Woodward and Potanin 2004).

3.8 A Paradigm Shift?

On an individual level, performance in surgery is like performance in sports but without a binary outcome. It cannot be reduced to winning or losing or even ranking. Much as we like to hear our patients suggest we are the 'top surgeon', I cannot see how this ranking is achieved or proved! Musicians' performance might be about winning or losing in a specific contest but assessment is generally more nuanced, more subjective more complex. It would be rather strange if a musical performance was judged purely by the accuracy of delivery as compared to the musical score and even worse if the first to finish said score 'won'. Virtuosity in music seems to contain many elements that are subjective and beyond the requirements of the music, it's not purely technical. Musical performance is perhaps closer to surgical performance but, as I mentioned earlier, the lack of complexity in surgical manoeuvres might simply level everyone with virtuosity impossible to tease out. Whatever the intangibles and tangibles I am inclined to agree with Potter Stewart in that, with regards to good surgery (as opposed to pornography), 'I know it when I see it'.

Having watched awe-inspiring performances in music and sport and having experienced the power of practice with my own musical renaissance, I can't help wondering if surgical performance could be improved if we could get closer to the paradigms of performance in music and sport. Spoiler alerts. In C.S Lewis' 'The Horse and His Boy', The horse Bree thinks he is running as fast as he can until the Lion appears and chases him. He then realises he can actually run much faster. Christian Bale's 'Batman' can only climb out of the pit *without* the rope, he has to be all in. There must be more? I will review and expose several aspects of the paradigm surgeons work within and explore what might push it in the direction of excellence.

3.9 Paradigm of Performance—Outcomes

From a patient's perspective, a surgeon's performance is often hidden with much judgement often simply placed on the scar or bedside manner! In ophthalmology my performance is more manifest than with many of the surgical specialities in that I have before and after scans of the retina in glorious detail and metrics of great importance to both the patient and me, their visual acuity. But even here so much still remains hidden. Clinical audit is required to continue to practice in the UK as part of annual appraisal. 'Gold standards' are set around very specific metrics and include common complications; they are very high-level and low resolution and perhaps simply signal safety rather than competence let alone excellence. (Hence my previous question of the 'Carat' of said 'Gold' standards). Nationally, results from clinical audit show very significant convergence of results with 95% of surgeons within the accepted ± 2 standard deviations. There is not enough nuance to assess surgical prowess on these results, they signal a 'threshold competence' rather than a 'core competence' and fail to demonstrate the type of excellence we see in sport and music. There will be no surgery category in the next Olympics.

3.10 Paradigm of Performance—Processes

Can we make the actual processes of surgery more visible and open to scrutiny or development? At one extreme, there are the conferences where 'live surgery' is performed in front of hundreds of surgeons, the ultimate in 'arena performance'. There are very mixed opinions about this. Having recordings of the surgery within the theatre does help to increase the visibility of surgery for those who have time to watch. Might this visibility drive performance or might it actually inhibit performance by increasing stress? If we go back to the Catastrophe model and IZOF in Chap. 1, some surgeons might like this additional stress and perform at a higher level others might struggle hence concerns over 'live surgery'. All surgeons have to have a degree of visibility in order to teach, does this drive performance? Most members of staff in theatre are too busy doing their individual jobs to watch a screen but there are two very important potential monitors of performance other than the surgeon. The scrub nurse and the trainee. The scrub nurse will assist with many surgeons and get an intuitive feel for how each surgeon performs as compared to others. The trainees have more specific technical knowledge of procedures than the scrub nurses and have some experience in performing them. Performing surgery is the only way to really understand surgery, until you attempt it, it is just too theoretical hence the limitations of imagery. Trainees get to watch many surgeons very closely and we all know they talk but extracting this powerful information is, how should I say it, delicate!

Practically, visibility will only be possible in specialities that use digital viewing systems in order to perform surgery and difficult for those using the naked eye unless body cams are worn! I am aware of a hospital that routinely records all eye surgery and all complications are reviewed. There are even significant consequences for being in the lower ranks at year end. Regardless, what I have found is recording my own surgery and then reviewing it is a useful tool for improvement. It allows review without the distractions and requirements of actual surgery. Even more powerful is training fellows and discussing cases, both yours and theirs. We will come to this again in 'Part III' with System 1 and 2 thinking.

3.11 Paradigm of Performance—Patient Experience

Musical performance is predominantly measured by the subjective and emotional responses of the audience. Athletic performance is judged more objectively. I have discussed the limitations of objective measurement in surgery as being generally 'threshold' or 'good enough'. We do, however, measure the subjective quality of patients' experience. Patient-reported outcomes (PROMs) are increasingly being used to assess the quality of care however, they cannot be too detailed, or else compliance falls, and so they tend to give very granular, low-resolution information. PROMS still operate on the 'threshold competence' level in my opinion and again represent 'good enough' not excellence. Patient experience in theatre is also very variable and difficult to assess especially (of course) when comparing general to local anaesthetic. In a small study in our unit, we showed that patient anxiety was subjectively lessened by music in theatre and by talking to the patient during surgery (Rufai et al. 2015). However, could an incredible bedside manner and great playlist cover up poor surgery? It is also interesting to note that in one study, the feature that was most correlated with patients recommending their surgeon to others was actually a personality characteristic, low neuroticism (Lanz et al. 2018). More on this in 'Part III'.

3.12 Pushing the Paradigm Yourself

We cannot achieve the level of comparison in performance of athletes or musicians and we cannot achieve their level of practice and training either. Music perhaps represents a closer paradigm to drive performance however lack of technical complexity might limit the concept of virtuosity in surgery, at least in 'Box 1' explored in 'Part I'. On speaking to a friend who works at a London Eye Hospital about this issue, she pointed out that the worlds of music and sport truly celebrate greatness but this does not happen in the NHS. This is very true, everyone is levelled off, resolution is to the level of acceptable or safe and so most performance remains under the radar. It is very difficult to shine and very easy to hide.

We are faced with a spectrum of interpretation in terms of our own paradigm of performance. At one end of the spectrum, nothing really matters. We are practising our golf swing, during a competition, in the dark, have no idea where the ball ends up and can make no useful changes to improve and the competition has no winners anyway. I don't like this position but can understand it. Moving away from fatalism along the spectrum, we may try to get better by measuring results as best we can and look for progress as I *think* I have. However, the results are too low resolution to actually detect any significant improvement and no one in our immediate environment cares anyway. It is rather frustrating that after 14 years as a consultant my outcomes remain about the same. They are also very similar to everyone else's, including my trainees! This is perhaps where most of us sit. We are stuck with 'threshold competence' with 95% of all surgeons achieving it and even if we find ourselves in the 5% outside the accepted competence level, we can claim the 'case mix' argument and wriggle out.

However, I believe the paradigm of performance can be 'pushed'. Why not attempt a magnification of the outcomes to get high resolution? Annual audit is low resolution, it's 'threshold competence'. Magnify; prospective audit, review as you go not at year end. This will focus attention on the results of each case allowing more ongoing reflection rather than the nebulous end-of-year review where the nuances of each case are lost. Magnify; review each case after surgery. What went well? What was suboptimal? Access your 'System 2' thinking ('Part III'). Magnify; review each section of the surgery, how was your 'micro-technique'? Draw from the chapter on Sports Psychology and set up 'mini-games' using goal setting theory. Split your surgery into multiple small sections, decide what perfect looks like for each section and score yourself as you go. Goal setting theory fits well with 'Lean processes' in 'Part II'. Look for marginal gains. Perfection is unlikely but you might get close at times.

3.13 Pushing the Paradigm—Coaches

It has struck me that in surgery we learn by imitation and teaching is limited by the consultant's experience and competence. I cannot train a fellow to do something I cannot do. Training (*not* learning) effectively stops at consultant level. Having a consultant 'buddy' who can intermittently review unedited random videos of surgery or at least your best and worst case of the season or actually sit in with you on a list is valuable. However, in order to truly push the paradigm here we need to think about the role of coaches. Coaches do not train by imitation; they apply knowledge and observation to direct the performer and invite them towards excellence. To protect our fragile egos, we need to imagine we are Usain Bolt and understand the person coaching us cannot beat us in a sprint but they have valuable insight to help us run even faster. The goal is somehow out there and objective not personal and must draw on all aspects of surgery, 'Part I' and beyond. To shift the paradigm will require enthusiasm. Be enthusiastic about your surgery and get someone else involved. 'Faithful are the wounds of a friend but the kisses of an enemy are deceitful'. (*Prov 27, 6*) Perhaps the surgical coach can become just that friend and we can strive together towards virtuosity in surgery.

3.14 Conclusion

Musicians offer insight into the performance of surgery in a manner that is less binary and more subjective than elite sports. Can we have virtuoso surgeons? I am not sure; surgery is perhaps not technical enough to allow for the wide distribution of technical ability required for the exception to emerge or perhaps musical virtuosity resides much more in 'Box 1' explored in 'Part I'. It is clear the dedication required for the musician to achieve virtuoso status is complete requiring a level of practice over a time period that cannot be matched in surgery. It also requires innate talent and intelligence and yet more practice. However, rather than give up and try to be good enough, with enthusiasm and the application of the tools discussed in 'Part I' the surgeon can at least push the paradigm and aim high.

3.15   To Try

Can you learn a new technical skill outside of surgery to understand the steps required to make progress and then see how you might apply it to your surgery?

Reflect on your own paradigm of performance. Do you find yourself saying 'I just…' when describing your surgery?

Marginal gains—can you break down to micro-technique and seek perfection?

What do you think a virtuoso surgeon would look like?

How might you develop and practice?

Would you employ a surgical coach, and what might they enable you to do?

References

Boyd T, Jung I, van Sickle K, Schwesinger W, Michalek J, Bingener J. Music experience influences laparoscopic skills performance. JSLS: J Soc Laparoendosc Surgeons, (n.d.);12(3), 292–4.

Czudek K. What does it take to become a professional pianist? n.d. https://Pianoground.Com/What-Does-It-Take-to-Become-a-Professional-Pianist/. Retrieved November 29, 2023, from https://pianoground.com/what-does-it-take-to-become-a-professional-pianist/

Ericsson KAKRTT-RC. The role of deliberate practice in the acquisition of expert performance. Psychol Rev. 1993;100(3):363–406.

Gladwell M. Outliers: The Story of Success. Penguin; 2009.

Lanz JJ, Gregory PJ, Menendez ME, Harmon L. Dr. Congeniality: Understanding the Importance of Surgeons' Nontechnical Skills Through 360° Feedback. J Surg Educ. 2018;75(4), 984–92. https://doi.org/10.1016/j.jsurg.2017.12.006.

Lynn R, Gault A. The relation of musical ability to general intelligence and the major primaries. Res Educ. 1986;36(1):59–64. https://doi.org/10.1177/003452378603600107.

Rufai SR, Mitchell BG, Farmer TD, Lash SC. Reducing anxiety during conscious surgery—a patient survey. Int J Surg. 2015;23:118–9. https://doi.org/10.1016/j.ijsu.2015.09.058.

Ruthsatz J, Detterman D, Griscom WS, Cirullo BA. Becoming an expert in the musical domain: it takes more than just practice. Intelligence. 2008;36(4):330–8. https://doi.org/10.1016/j.intell.2007.08.003.

Spiteri AV, Aggarwal R, Kersey TL, Sira M, Benjamin L, Darzi AW, Bloom PA. Development of a virtual reality training curriculum for phacoemulsification surgery. Eye. 2014;28(1):78–84. https://doi.org/10.1038/eye.2013.211.

Vouhé PR. The surgeon and the musician☆. Eur J Cardiothorac Surg. 2011;39(1):1–5. https://doi.org/10.1016/j.ejcts.2010.11.046.

Woodward C, Potanin F. Winning!: The path to Rugby World Cup Glory. Hodder and Stoughton Ltd.; 2004.

Part II
The 'What' of Surgery

Introduction

'Part II' will explore the planning of surgery and the barriers to our 'best laid plans'. It is in this box we begin to see the style and approach of the surgeon reveal itself. The cornerstone chapter will focus on applying Toyota car manufacturing, or more specifically, 'Lean' manufacturing processes to the practice of surgery. I will explore the concepts of 'Kaizen', 'right first time', and the elimination of 'Muda' or waste. I will apply the seven wastes to surgery and explore their utility in the pursuit of great surgery. Surgeons improve by taking responsibility. If everything is the surgeon's fault, they can learn, if nothing is their fault, they are powerless. This will be explored in a chapter on 'Locus of Control'. We all want to succeed but perhaps, even more so, we do not want to fail (Part III). Fear of Failure is the most common reason I would stray from the 'Lean' path and I will argue there has never been a worse time to fail in history.

Chapter 4
Lean Surgery—What Can We Learn from Toyota?

The first stage of improving efficiency in surgery is to stop doing nothing. The second stage is to stop repeating things and the third stage is to stop doing certain things. Finally be dissatisfied and circle back.

—Stephen Lash

Abstract I will review the key aspects of 'Lean' production, specifically the seven wastes, and map them onto surgical processes. The wastes include motion, inventory, waiting, defects, overprocessing, overproduction and transportation. Some map onto surgery better than others and there is some overlap. How do we practice 'Kaizen' or continuous improvement and aim to get surgical manoeuvres right first time? Having learned about the wastes you will be encouraged to review your own surgery in the light of these and explore how you might develop your technique in a 'Lean' direction improving your efficiency and reducing errors.

Keywords Lean production · Seven wastes · Kaizen · Taiichi Ohno · Continuous improvement · Reflective practice · Surgeon's performance · Surgical decision-making

4.1 Introduction

In 'Part I' I focussed on improving 'performance' in the surgical field, in the moment of surgery, and reviewed evidence from Sports Psychology, simulators, pilots and musicians to support this aim. I discussed what could be learned from elite athletes in terms of mental preparation and execution under stress. PMST was applied to surgery and the evidence was reviewed with some positive avenues to explore and implement. I examined the utility of simulators as a tool for practice and found they work very well at the beginning of the learning curve, reducing real-world complications, but sadly lacking in utility at higher levels of performance. I also explored how we might 'push the paradigm' of performance to get closer to the elites and virtuosos in sport and music. The current culture seems one of adequacy and safety rather than true excellence but we do not currently have the tools to train or rehearse as effectively as the athletes and musicians do. It's hard to shine and easy to hide in the milieu of 'adequate' but *you* will know. Be enthusiastic.

This next perspective moves out of 'Box 1' (explored in Part I) and into a bigger box, 'Box 2' (to be explored in this section, Part II). 'Box 2' heavily influences the first 'box'. How can we organise our surgery? The perspective in 'Part II' centres on an assumption that we can apply Toyota 'Lean' car manufacturing processes to surgery. There is no evidence base for this specific application. We are truly in the sand so I would remove your shoes to avoid getting irritating bits stuck in your socks. This chapter invites the reader to explore the concepts with an open mind and take from them what works. Lean has been applied to Emergency Departments and the running of medical services with numerous publications but not, as far as I am aware, to the actual *practice* of surgery. I will start with a brief history of car manufacturing and the emergence of 'Lean', an academic term applied to the Toyota Production System or TPS. Many of you will remember the 'Japanese invasion' of the car industry in the 1980s. This is the story behind that. It turned car manufacturing on its head and although it will not revolutionise surgery, I do hope its application will be beneficial in improving skills and outcomes. I will apply Lean principles to surgery with the main thrust the elimination of 'Muda' or waste. Next, I will look at some of the potential barriers to implementing Lean surgery notably 'locus of control' and 'failure'. I will review society's view of failure over the last 2000 years and come to the conclusion that there has never been a worse time in history to fail! I will also explore failure within the culture of the airline industry and surgery and finally the self. I hate failure more than I like success ('Part III') and if I am not careful it can change the way I operate. I can end up treating myself rather than the patient. The pain of failure can be lessened by pushing responsibility outside of yourself but there are consequences for learning and progression. I heard the story of an enigmatic gastric surgeon on a post-operative ward round who was reviewing a patient following failed surgery. He took her by the hand, patted it gently and reassured her empathetically, 'You must not blame yourself dear!'.

You may see no potential benefits in applying Lean principles to surgery or you may feel the principles are just obvious. Some of this might be personality, which we will explore in 'Part III' or how you have been trained. Regardless, read on with an open mind and feel the sand between your toes, a pleasant experience, rather than sand in your shoes, a rather irritating experience.

4.2 Lean Production—What Has Toyota Got to Do with Surgery?

Automobile production has evolved through several stages over the last century and a half, each improving the quality *and* quantity of cars produced. 1672 saw the production of the first steam-powered vehicle capable of human transport. Carl

Benz is widely accepted to be the 'father' of the modern automobile with a gasoline-powered engine produced in 1886. Both vehicles were the result of 'craft' production. Craft production is time consuming and very expensive hence only around 100 cars were made per year. Each car was built to the exact specifications of the customer, there was incredible variety. It was truly a customer-oriented market. Henry Ford introduced mass production in 1903 shifting to a more product-oriented view of the market although aiming to serve a mass consumer market. 'You can have any colour as long as it's black'. In phase 1, a single fitter would assemble the entire car. This task cycle took 514 minutes. In 1908 he achieved perfect part interchangeability enabling each fitter to work on a specific part. The fitter remained in one spot whilst the car moved along a 'production line'. By the end of 1913 the assembly line was created and the average task cycle for the assembler reduced from 514 to 2.3 minutes. (Womack et al. 1990) Taylorism or scientific management, is a theory that analyses and synthesises work flows. Taylor began presenting his theory during the late nineteenth century with peak influence around 1910 and he introduced some powerful, now ubiquitous, themes including logic, rationality, empiricism, work ethic, efficiency, elimination of waste and standardisation of best practices. With each assembler performing a limited set of tasks they became very competent at each, more accurate, more efficient and much faster. With Ford's mass production, costs reduced as did the time to produce each car. Volumes increased and cars became affordable. By the early 1930s over 30 million vehicles were produced and sold all over the world with Ford, Chrysler and General Motors (The Big Three) dominating the market.

However, there were problems with this mass production model. The separation of labour in the workforce resulted in 'gaps' through which errors could occur. A design engineer created the blueprint for the assembly line solving the mathematical problems inherent in this process in terms of the time required for each section and the order of assembly. However, strict control of the supply chain, ordering and storage of parts was required for the line to function as well as the coordination of many workers each working at a single station. Many other staff were required including repair men to refurbish tools, quality specialists to check the work and rework men at the end of the line to repair and make good earlier errors and omissions (Which might be buried beneath layers of panel work and upholstery). Matters were made worse by the 'move the metal' mentality which meant only the foreman could stop the line. Pay was determined by production quotas, there was pressure to keep the line moving. As a result, many of the cars sold to the public were defective.

For various reasons this model of mass production did not work in Japan. There was a lack of immigrant workers prepared to perform the soul-destroying repetitive tasks required. The market was smaller and required a more diverse offering from luxury cars and small run around city cars to trucks. Between 1925 and 1936 the Big Three dominated the Japanese market supplying 200,000 vehicles whilst Japanese companies produced only 12,000. Japan needed to think differently and the 'Toyota way' was born.

Toyota engineers Taiichi Ohno and Eiji Toyoda developed their process for manufacturing cars and called it the Toyota Production System or TPS. The term 'Lean' was coined by John Krafcik in 1988 following his analysis of 37 assembly plants and was later used by James Womack in his book 'The Machine That Changed the World' (Womack et al. 1990) Womack and his team observed many differences between the American and Japanese plants. In the American plants there was lots of space between production lines with piles of inventory filling the aisles. In the Japanese plants there was very little space which facilitated face-to-face contact and there were no piles of inventory as it was supplied to the line 'just in time'. TPS valued continuous improvement (Kaizen) and every worker was able to 'stop the line' if a problem occurred, not just the foreman. Each worker was encouraged to improve the system when a fault was found by asking the 'five whys'. The net result was getting the car 'right first time' so no need for a rework area. Another important part of lean production was the elimination of waste (Muda). This waste was defined with respect to the end-user or customer. Lean was born out of necessity to deliver a competitive advantage over the US car industry and it was highly successful with the subsequent domination of multiple international car markets from the early 70s, 'The Japanese Invasion'. Lean has now spread to multiple sectors including healthcare.

Can I apply these Lean processes to surgery? In a similar way to the process of car manufacturing, I believe surgery can be viewed as a 'production line' made up of a series of steps or surgical manoeuvres applied to the patient in a particular sequence to arrive at the completion of the treatment. Hopefully, as in Lean, there is a good outcome, minimal defects and efficient use of the limited resources available including time, equipment and staff. I want to apply some of the important aspects underpinning Lean including—'Kaizen' (Continuous improvement), 'right first time' and the elimination of 'Muda' (Waste).

4.3 The Elimination of Waste (Muda)

Muda is one of the three types of deviation from the optimal allocation of resources. Muda means 'futility', 'uselessness' or 'wastefulness'. Muda is applied with specific reference to the end-user and might be non-value adding but of use (Type I) or simply waste (Type II). For example, safety testing a part does not add value but is required to ensure a safe product for the customer (Type 1). Type II waste should be eliminated.

There are seven forms of waste and I will try to apply these to surgery and see if this 'lens' sheds any new light on surgical technique. Not all wastes map well onto surgery with some overlap. The underlying assumption here is that the improvements seen in car manufacturing following the introduction of Lean will translate into improvements in patients' surgical care. Improvements in car manufacturing included better utilisation of resources, less errors, more efficient production and greater volumes. Surgically, I would hope to see better utilisation of resources, less complications, more efficient surgery and more patients treated per list. Treating more patients on a list will result in additional benefits to the people who are currently on waiting lists or even waiting to be seen. These 'people', who are not yet 'patients', often have deteriorating pathology and likely worsening final outcomes when they do eventually

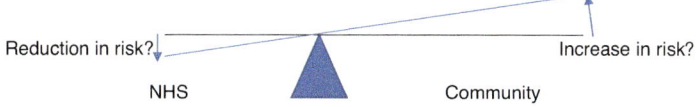

Fig. 4.1 Risk see-saw—where is the fulcrum?

get into surgery. I think as surgeons it is easy to lose sight of these people, they are not our responsibility yet.

Lean is driven by the customer. As an important aside, if the 'customer' of health-care is the general population, then I believe that what we are seeing currently in the NHS is an increase in bureaucracy and protocol-driven care in order to, I would argue, incrementally improve safety *within the system.* That means more time taken per patient and less time available for new patients. The risk may be reducing in ever-decreasing increments *within the system* but increasing significantly *outside the system*, like a see-saw. I am not sure where the fulcrum of this see-saw sits but I suspect it is not central and small reductions in risk within the system might be magnifying risk outside the system. (Fig. 4.1) If lean can allow more patients to be treated per list this will be good for 'patients' within the system and good for the 'people' outside.

In the following section a brief explanation of each form of waste in manufacturing will be presented and a surgical application discussed. There will be tasks to try at the end of the chapter.

4.4 Motion

Motion includes movements of people or machines which are more complicated or prolonged than absolutely necessary and further, may cause harm to equipment or people.

Excessive movement in terms of repetition and / or magnitude within the surgical field will increase the risk of inadvertent tissue damage. Wasted movement that does not achieve what it sets out to achieve, will prolong surgery times which may contribute to other complications from anaesthetic to Intraoperative to post-operative. In the ideal scenario, the 'intention to execution' ratio for each manoeuvre is 1:1, no repetition, no excessive movement, right first time. One review found that complications rates increased by 14% for every thirty minutes additional surgical time. (Cheng et al. 2018) Duration of surgery was found to be a risk factor in post-cataract surgery endophthalmitis (Garcia-Arumi et al. 2007). But thinking beyond the individual patient, longer surgery means less surgeries performed on each list which might result in longer waiting lists and the complications that occur with delayed treatment as well as the poor utilisation of expensive and limited resources, a theatre and its staff and a surgeon.

4.5   Inventory

Inventory should be sufficient to fulfil customer needs. Inventory should be sufficient to carry out the required tasks and no more. Excessive inventory kept 'Just in case' should be eliminated.

I am not going to cover procurement and ordering of equipment in the supply chain although that is a very appropriate area in terms of 'just in time' processes. In applying inventory to surgery, I would argue that inventory can be viewed from two perspectives, physical and procedural. The physical equipment and disposables required to do the surgery can be a source of waste. Having everything you might need open is a potential waste of resources financially but it may also clutter the surgical space making the job of the scrub nurse more difficult and interfering with the teamwork required for efficient surgery. At a procedural level, inventory can be seen as the micro-surgical interventions selected in each case, the toolbox of techniques used during surgery. In this definition each step performed should be just sufficient to achieve the end goal and no more, it should be 'right first time'. I see this definition of inventory most often violated in what I call the 'Snowball technique' which may also include other wastes.

4.6   The Snowball Technique

I will use an example from ophthalmology but you will have examples in whatever surgery you perform. A trainee will perform an additional (in my opinion unnecessary) manoeuvre—excess inventory. I will ask why they have performed this and they will reply with a 'just in case' type argument often fuelled by the 'availability heuristic' (the one that went wrong- See 'Part III') and also failing to do the first step 'right first time', a key principle of lean. The most common example I see is in the formation of the main incision and the paracentesis (side incision), in cataract surgery. The keratome is passed to the surgeon and the main incision is formed. The keratome is returned to the scrub nurse (motion waste, risk of damage to the keratome and the scrub nurse and the surgeon—I have witnessed all of these!). A viscoelastic (a viscous fluid used to fill and support the surgical space) is then passed to the surgeon and injected into the anterior chamber and passed back (more motion waste). The keratome is then returned to the surgeon and the paracentesis is made and the keratome passes back and forth again (more motion waste and risk) When asked 'why' the trainee will often recount a time when the anterior chamber collapsed (not doing the first incision 'right first time' plus an availability heuristic—the one that went wrong), 'risk aversion' further drives this behaviour ('Part III'). Hence the second and third manoeuvres simply add more 'snow' to the snowball which, over time, will continue to grow as other measures are added 'just in case', resulting in an excessive technique (Overproduction waste see later). It's very hard to stop doing something in surgery. Forming both sections with the keratome in one pass, without the anterior chamber collapsing, is more in keeping with Lean.

4.7   Waiting

Waiting is usually caused by the asynchrony of two or more interdependent processes. The hole is drilled but the bolt is not ready hence the production line comes to a standstill. Removing waiting makes the process more efficient and cost effective which saves both time and money.

Surgically I see two aspects to this waste. The first is when a surgeon simply stops for no apparent reason, the second is something unrelated to surgery is happening and so surgery stops. If nothing is happening then the surgeon needs to reflect on why this is. Are they waiting on instruments in which case did they inform the scrub nurse ahead of time what would be required? Are they unsure of the next step or are they thinking about what they have just done? 'Flow' has been shown to be an important and extremely beneficial state in many activities, including surgery, and is achieved when concentration is focussed on the present moment (Csikszentmihalyi 1990) Alternatively, something is happening but it is unrelated to the actual surgical task directly like readjusting the microscope, readjusting the seating or adjusting the volume on the music. In this case I would suggest thorough preparation before surgery commences and good communication with the team during surgery to avoid this wait. However, 'nothing happening' may be quite appropriate at times. Something has changed, a complication or an abnormal response to a surgical manoeuvre in which case nothing is *the best thing* to be happening such that the next move is the best solution to the ensuing problem. Surgeons often compound complications if they are not careful, see the 'defects' section below. One of the first tasks I offer to trainees is to record their surgery and do a time and motion study and identify all the times nothing is happening, it is significant.

4.8   Defects

The waste of defects includes quality errors. If these are ignored, they often cause more expense and time to fix at a later date and may lead to failure of the product with the customer. This was seen in the US car manufacturing plants where many of the cars required reworking in the rework areas at the end of the lines and customers found high levels of unreliability.

Surgically this is critical. I believe the surgeon creates most of their own problems and these have a habit of compounding and amplifying. I often see this effect when an apparently minor issue at the start of a procedure is not dealt with and rapidly gives birth to issues of ever-increasing severity and difficulty. An example might be as simple as poor draping of the eye with the eyelashes uncovered and protruding into the surgical field. This reduces the surgeon's view which can result in a more serious error and so on. Issues should be dealt with as they arise to prevent amplification and further, as in the TPS, the surgeon should ask 'Why' this has happened and correct it.

4.9 Overprocessing

Overprocessing waste is putting more work into producing the product than the customer values.

Surgically I see this most commonly express itself in the 'snowball technique' at the level of specific manoeuvres in the surgical process. With the snowball technique years of small complications and the resultant 'added preventative actions' build up resulting in an excessive technique. It is very difficult to stop doing something you have always done, to take away from a process, even to delete a repeated photo in your photo library. Overprocessing can involve several of the other wastes including motion, inventory and defects as detailed previously. They all become hidden in the excess.

4.10 Overproduction

This can lead to other wastes but can hide them making it all very difficult to untangle. This waste occurs when production exceeds customer requirements, which leads to high levels of inventory.

Overproduction can be related to inexperience with experienced surgeons generally less likely to intervene and overtreat, but not always. Experienced surgeons have more confidence than those starting out. I saw it in myself in the first year of my consultant post where I was scared to fail and tended to overtreat 'just to be sure'. Many other factors might contribute to overproduction and we will discuss these in 'Part III'. An interesting philosophical question to ask yourself about your approach to surgery is do you work 'with the grain of nature' or is everything a 'battle'? This ethos is often revealed in comments made during surgery. Listen out for 'If it's going to go wrong it will!' or 'that should be fine!'. If it's a battle then you are more likely to be prone to overproduction.

Common examples in ophthalmology include the gas tamponade used in the eye after surgery for macular holes. Treatment for macular holes started in the early 1990s with a gas used in the eye that lasted two months. The patient cannot see or fly with gas in the eye. Remember, 'Lean' focusses on what is of value to the end-user and losing full sight for two months is not to be underestimated and unlikely to be welcomed by the patient. However, as with other surgical interventions, they tend to be appropriately cautious at the start, the 'precautionary principle', and become less so and more 'Lean' over time with advances in technology, better understanding of the disease and clinical audit of results. Some surgeons now advocate using air with small holes, which lasts a week, and others a gas that lasts two weeks, five weeks or two months for larger holes. As a result of this wide accepted practice, the surgeon's attitude to failure and risk may push them to use a longer-acting gas than another surgeon resulting in prolonged poor sight and an inability to travel for the patient. I will cover 'Fear of Failure in 'Part II' combined with the very powerful heuristics in 'Part III'.

The other example I use with my trainees is in treating retinal detachments where the surgeon needs to close all the breaks with cryotherapy or laser. Treatment results in scarring. In this scenario, I use an analogy that the first procedure is like walking into a grassy field to deal with a single molehill. If they walk across the field, dig up the molehill and walk away if another molehill appears they will spot it easily and can fix it. If they pile in with a JCB digger the first time, the field is carnage and if another mole hill pops up it will be difficult to spot. If you are going to fail then fail well. Fear of failure is a big driver to overproduction and overprocessing and the surgeon ends up treating themselves more than the patient.

There is no easy analysis other than continuous review of your own cases with honest reflection, including an element of peer review and clinical audit, to help contribute some 'objective' data to the process. Honest review of your attitude to surgery can also be of benefit. Is surgery a battle or is the body actually 'on your side!'?

4.11   Transportation

Transportation of materials requires time and incurs a cost. If the movement of materials does not directly correspond to some value-adding process then it represents a waste of time and money and may result in damage to the objects being transported.

Surgically this is similar to the movement waste and would encourage the surgeon to minimise tissue manipulation and movement.

Beyond 'Muda', other concepts are important in lean processes, Mura, Muri and Kaizen.

4.12   Mura

Mura is imbalance or inconsistency in operation. Surgery is not entirely like a manufacturing process as essentially it is one biological system intervening in another through instruments and machines. A lot can happen in terms of variability and response to each surgical manoeuvre unlike the more consistent nature of a purely physical engineering processes. However, the aim in surgery should be consistency in the procedure with every patient. Of course, variability in anatomy and complications will lead to deviations but these should be the exception. This is perhaps supported by the observations I made in the section on learning curves. As trainees progress through their training their cases are performed more quickly and more consistently with less variation in time. As we get more experienced, we should naturally tend to move away from Mura.

4.13 Muri

Muri is the overburdening of equipment, employees, or processes by requiring them to operate too fast, with too much effort, or for longer than equipment designs permit and good workforce management allow.

It is easy to see how this applies to public healthcare systems with finite resources dealing with ever-increasing demands. However, in surgery specifically, muri can occur when surgical technique is not lean. Longer surgeries are tiring and can result in damage to the surgeon. We see this all too often in Ophthalmology with back issues very common (Venkatesh and Kumar 2017) Even a lean technique can come under pressure when lists are overbooked or the demands on balancing finish time with patient experience and teaching opportunities for the juniors become a complex conundrum.

4.14 Kaizen

Kaizen is derived from two words meaning change (Kai) and good (Zen). In this sense Kaizen simply means change for the better but it should also be continuous. Kaizen as a method or business tool is comprised of a trio of elements. Kaizen or continuous improvement is sought in every small step by constantly challenging the work environment and looking to eliminate Muda, Mura and Muri. 'Kaikaku' is a radical or revolutionary change from innovation or disruption and may be required where small incremental changes are not sufficient to solve the problem. And finally, 'sustainability' with each improvement embedded in new standards.

Kaizen is particularly powerful when every employee in the organisation has the ability to identify and eliminate waste in their work. In order to deliver this, staff need to feel empowered and able to contribute and comment. The airline industry had to address the hierarchy issues with their 'Crew Resource Management' in the cockpit after failures led to crashes. As we saw in 'Part I' this has worked extremely well and is firmly embedded into the culture. Similar moves have been attempted in the theatre environment as lack of teamworking is often the cause of medical errors. However, specifically with regard to surgery, I think it is most usefully applied in a personal way with prospective audit, reflective practice and collaboration and honest discussion with other colleagues both senior and junior.

4.15   Conclusion

There are many aspects to surgery that map well on to the processes of Lean car manufacturing and the observations feel useful. Intuitively, accurate efficient surgery should be better for patients and enable more patients to be treated more efficiently. In my childhood I remember watching the 'Generation Game' where an expert would perform a task in front of the participating family like making pasta. They would be slick and fast and 'Lean' it would look effortless. Then a family member would 'have a go' and chaos would ensue. Lean looks fantastic, it looks expert but in reality, it would be impossible to do a study to prove it.

4.16   Tasks to Try

4.16.1   Motion/Transportation

Task—Record a common surgery and review it (playing at fast forward often exacerbates the movements). Are there excessive movements? Are there unnecessary movements? Are there repeated movements? Can you refine your movements and reduce them? Can you achieve the same surgical end for the specific task better, with less movement, less tissue disruption? Do you need all the movements to achieve the same end (Snowball technique see below).

4.16.2   Inventory

Task—Record a common surgery and review it. Review each step and ask why? Discuss with another surgeon who may approach the surgery differently to you. Discuss with an experienced surgeon and be aware of heuristics (Part III). Review the literature but be aware of the limitations of evidence-based medicine in surgery as ultimately it is 'in your hands' not the published author or their teams' hands. Can you reduce your inventory?

4.16.3   Waiting

Task—Record a common surgery and review it. Are there periods of time when nothing is happening? Why is nothing happening? Are you trying to remember what is next or going over what you have just done? Are you attending to something other than the surgery? Do you need to attend to this or can a member of the team attend to this? Asking the scrub nurse to change setting on the machine results in a delay that could be avoided if settings can be changed on the foot pedal by the surgeon. Had something gone wrong, in which case nothing was the right thing to do.

4.16.4 Defects

Task—Record a common surgery and review it. Review a case with a complication. Can you trace the complication back to its cause? Ask why repeatedly until you get to the root. Learn as much as you can from this process and apply it to future surgeries. Avoid an 'external locus of control' mindset (To be covered soon!). If it is not your fault you are powerless to change and cannot get better.

4.16.5 Overproduction/Overprocessing

Task—Record a common surgery and review it. Note down your micro-technique, each individual step that makes up a small section of surgery. Review these steps, are they all necessary? Review each section, is each necessary and what does excellent look like and how do you compare? Are you performing any 'just in case' manoeuvres? Do you need to do these? Sometimes these are necessary even though they do not add to the patient's outcome directly (Type 1). Have you performed each manoeuvre right first time? Are you making up for poor technique by adding stages? How did you arrive at your technique and can you assist other surgeons who do it differently to you or your trainer? Do you need to practice specific manoeuvres in a dry lab/ simulator (Apply Taylorism and improve efficiency and accuracy by repetition)?

References

Cheng H, Clymer JW, Po-Han Chen B, Sadeghirad B, Ferko NC, Cameron CG, Hinoul P. Prolonged operative duration is associated with complications: a systematic review and meta-analysis. J Surg Res. 2018;229:134–44. https://doi.org/10.1016/j.jss.2018.03.022.
Csikszentmihalyi M. Flow: the psychology of optimal experience. Harper and Row; 1990.
Garcia-Arumi J, Fonollosa A, Sararols L, Fina F, Martínez-Castillo V, Boixadera A, Zapata MA, Campins M. Topical anesthesia: possible risk factor for endophthalmitis after cataract extraction. J Cataract Refract Surg. 2007;33(6):989–92. https://doi.org/10.1016/j.jcrs.2007.02.030.
Venkatesh R, Kumar S. Back pain in ophthalmology: national survey of Indian ophthalmologists. Indian J Ophthalmol. 2017;65(8):678. https://doi.org/10.4103/ijo.IJO_344_17.
Womack JP, Jones DT, Roos D. The machine that changed the world: the story of lean production. Harper Perennial; 1990.

Chapter 5
Locus of Control—What We Can Learn from Taking Responsibility?

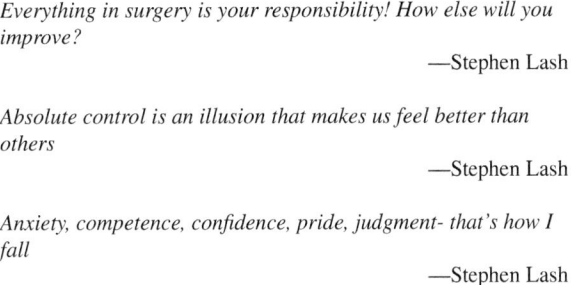

Everything in surgery is your responsibility! How else will you improve?

—Stephen Lash

Absolute control is an illusion that makes us feel better than others

—Stephen Lash

Anxiety, competence, confidence, pride, judgment- that's how I fall

—Stephen Lash

Abstract In this short chapter I want to focus on one barrier to 'Lean' surgery but also, I believe, a barrier to any good surgery or even skill in general, 'Locus of control'(LOC). The great surgeons I have met tend towards a high internal LOC and thus they tend to take responsibility for what happens in theatre. People with a high external LOC tend to blame external circumstances. I think it is important that 'everything is your fault' as a surgeon or else how can you make progress? However, in some respects, this barrier to Lean might also be a barrier to developing a culture accepting of failure, which I will discuss next.

Keywords Locus of control (LOC) · Surgeon's performance · Surgical decision-making · Multidimensional health locus of control scale (MHLC) · Lean surgery · Health psychology · Surgery improvement · Proactive focus · Reactive focus

The concept of 'Locus of control' (LOC) was developed by Julian Rotter in the 1950s and 1960s (Rotter 1966) He developed a questionnaire to determine the degree to which a person believes they are in control of their life as opposed to the subject of external events. The concept has generated much research in the field of psychology although there is debate over whether a global or domain-specific approach is more useful. As far as I am aware there is no domain-specific assessment for LOC in surgery and so I will apply the more global approaches. Even in my own life there are things I do where I am more than happy to go with the flow but others where I could be accused of being a control freak. Surgery is the latter for me.

It is important to note that Rotter cautioned that LOC represents a spectrum, rather than a dichotomy, from an internal LOC (I) to an external LOC (E). 'I's' tend to believe that their hard work leads to success and favourable outcomes and that every action has a consequence. 'E's' tend to believe that outcomes are more attributed to external circumstances that are beyond their control. 'I's' tend to have a high level of need for achievement because if they believe their efforts can be rewarded and they believe they have agency in achieving their goal, a virtuous circle is set up, more effort more reward, etc. However, failure for 'I's' can be difficult and taken very personally. There is also some evidence that internal LOC increases over time peaking in middle age and then shifting externally as retirement progresses which makes intuitive sense when you think of children and the elderly (Gatz and Karel 1993) Upbringing can influence locus of control with a lower socioeconomic upbringing more likely to result in an External LOC (Schneewind 1995).

LOC has been utilised in the area of health psychology. One example is the Multidimensional Health Locus of Control Scale (MHLC) (Wallston et al. 1978) This suggests that health may be attributed to three sources, 'internal factors' such as lifestyle, and 'external factors' or 'powerful others', such as doctors and 'luck or chance'. People who tend towards 'luck or chance' are very difficult to help as they will not take responsibility (lifestyle) or trust the powerful others (doctors). In the surgical field I see this manifest most often in the surgical debrief and I suspect that 'I's' make better progress as surgeons than 'E's'. For example, listen to these debriefs following a difficult case.

Trainee 1. 'I am not very used to this theatre and the lighting was not great. I do not have my own settings on the microscope or the pedals yet so I was a bit slow. The drape was not very good and the patient kept moving making surgery very difficult'.

Trainee 2. 'I am not very used to this theatre so I came in early to check settings, and although I am not used to these settings, I think they can be improved over time. I will contact the rep. I really mucked up the drape, I did not dry the lids very well and struggled to get the clip in. The patient was quite mobile and I think I should have used a different anaesthetic approach to reduce this and more communication with the patient during the procedure might have helped reduce anxiety. I have work to do but am looking forward to improving!'.

Granted, these are somewhat exaggerated but I have heard both these types of reflections many times. I find an external LOC in a trainee a bit of a trigger. To be honest, I often react with an external locus statement and then deliberately and quickly follow this with an internal one to ensure I do not fall foul of my own trigger! Jung would suggest that 'Understanding what irritates us about others can also be vital to understanding ourselves'. The problem with having an external LOC in surgery is that there is no way to improve as nothing is your fault. A high Internal LOC puts you in a powerful position to improve because everything is your fault!

It is a spectrum worth some reflection. Where might you reside and can you push yourself gently towards an Internal LOC? Reviewing your surgery after each case is important. What went well and what went badly and why? What could *you* do differently next time? In terms of Lean, a high internal LOC will be synergistic. Lean requires a constant refinement of micro-technique to deliver Kaizen and eliminate Muda. It is synergistic with elements of the Sports Psychology discussed in 'Part I'. Goal setting and imagery require a detailed review of surgery at the micro-level to maximise the benefits of these techniques.

In his book 'The Seven Habits of Highly Effective People', Covey introduced his concept of the 'circle of concern' and 'circle of influence', the latter smaller and sitting within the former (Covey 1989). He suggests that a 'proactive focus' results in an enlargement of the circle of influence into the circle of concern however, a 'reactive focus' result in shrinkage of this circle with less influence and more concern. A central circle of control has been added by others although the more experienced I get the less sure I am of what actual control I really have in surgery. Herein lies the paradox with my argument. I argue for an internal locus of *control* but then state we have no real control! For example, we can control our movements in the surgical field but as we saw in 'Part I', physiological stress can result in physical effects limiting this control, notably tremor, and tissues can respond differently to the same rehearsed movement of the same instrument in our hands. This reflects the limitations of viewing surgery simply in 'Part I'. Perhaps we should really aim for a high 'internal locus of influence'. With time and experience a 'proactive focus', perhaps more likely in someone with a high Internal LOC, will result in enlargement of the circle of influence which also becomes more stable freeing up mental bandwidth to survey the outer circle of concern, where imminent curve balls and complications lie in wait. In this way the surgeon can attend to this dark outer circle and make plans to avoid the complication that might subsequently manifest. This overlaps with system thinking which is 'Part III' territory. The circles of influence and concern should also extend beyond the surgical field into the theatre in order to provide an environment suitable for excellent surgery. For example, simply playing music may improve your physical performance, team function and patient experience as we saw in 'Part I' (Allen 1994). Become an influencer of circumstance not a victim. However, it may be that having a profession full of people with a high internal LOC might result in a shift in culture to one intolerant of failure? I will explore this further in the next chapter but if we immediately blame ourselves for failure why would we not immediately blame others for theirs?

5.1 To Try

Reflect on a case that has gone well and one that had complications. Why did they go the way they did? Were you really in control?

What was under your 'control' and what was outside your 'control'? What was within your sphere of influence? What was in your sphere of concern and could it have been brought into the sphere of influence? How?

If a complication appeared outside your control ask the five whys from TPS, can you trace it back to a decision you made that if made differently might have prevented the complication? Did you ignore an issue in your sphere of concern (waste of defects)? Could you have increased your sphere of influence? How?

After reflecting on an aspect of surgery, play the scenario through again in your mind (Imagery) and rehearse interventions thus increasing your sphere of influence.

References

Allen K. Effects of music on cardiovascular reactivity among surgeons. JAMA: J Am Med Assoc. 1994;272(11), 882. https://doi.org/10.1001/jama.1994.03520110062030

Covey, S.R. The seven habits of highly effective people. (Free Press, Ed.); 1989.

Gatz M, Karel MJ. Individual change in perceived control over 20 years. Int J Behav Dev. 1993;16(2):305–22. https://doi.org/10.1177/016502549301600211.

Rotter JB. Generalized expectancies for internal versus external control of reinforcement. Psychol Monogr Gen Appl. 1966;80(1):1–28. https://doi.org/10.1037/h0092976.

Schneewind KA (1995) Impact of family processes on control beliefs. In: Self-efficacy in changing societies. Cambridge University Press, pp. 114–148. https://doi.org/10.1017/CBO9780511152 7692.006

Wallston KA, Strudler Wallston B, DeVellis R. Development of the multidimensional health locus of control (MHLC) scales. Health Educ Monogr. 1978;6(1):160–70. https://doi.org/10.1177/ 109019817800600107.

Chapter 6
Barriers to Lean Surgery—What can we Learn from Failure?

Surgical failure is a reminder there is more to do- are we nearly there yet? Not really!

—Stephen Lash

I was very scared of failure early on. I still don't like it but have tried to do it better every year

—Stephen Lash

Learning from mistakes is absolutely essential, and I find it easier and much more comfortable to learn from other people's

—Stephen Lash

Abstract When it comes to practising surgery and especially 'Lean' surgery, fear of failure plays a critical role for me and, I suspect, many other surgeons. It is certainly the factor that is most likely to encourage me off the 'Lean' path and lead me to overtreat and doubt my own judgements. I end up treating myself not the patient. But why is failing so terrible? In this section I will argue that there has never been a worse time in history to fail. Society won't forget it; surgeons fear it and our self-esteem forbids it. We need to learn to fail and fail well.

Keywords Lean surgery · Fear of failure · Surgeon's performance · Surgical decision-making · Surgery improvement · Spectrum of failure · Surgeon's responsibility

Our understanding of failure ultimately sits within our society's view of failure within the current culture. This has changed significantly over time as I will discuss. The concept of failure also differs between cultures and so I will limit my thoughts to my own, current, Western culture. The healthcare profession sits as an entity within this culture and is heavily influenced by it. There is much ongoing comparison between healthcare and aviation however, the 'no blame culture' of the airline industry is firmly embedded whereas in medicine and specifically surgery, less so even though we sit within the same Western culture. Why the difference? The interview with The Captain provided great insight into the differences and was striking. Finally,

Fig. 6.1 Failure nest

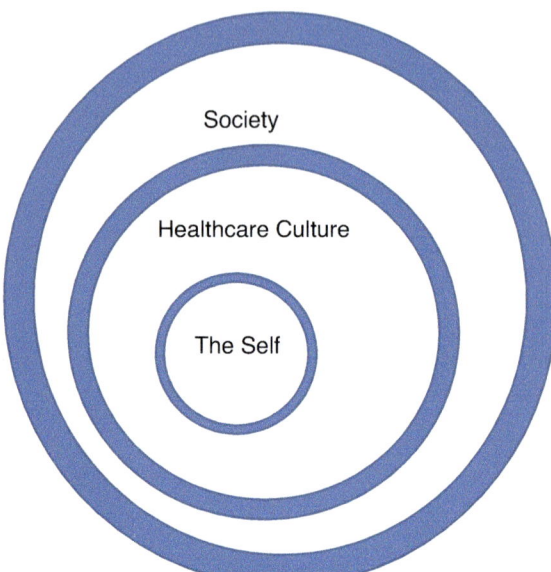

the understanding of failure sits within the view of the self which is again heavily influenced by society at large. Our society increasingly puts the 'self' at the centre of the entire universe. Failure of the self can be catastrophic, suicide the ultimate consequence, but it also manifests in low grade anxiety and depression which are all on the increase sadly. I am keen to explore these three concentric subcultures, self, profession and society and see what barriers might be revealed to embracing failure as a positive driver for good facilitating better surgery and improving patient outcomes *(*Fig. 6.1*)*.

6.1 A Personal Reflection on Failure in Surgery

In my first year as a consultant, I had the highest success rate of any year since for retinal detachment repairs. However, as I have reflected on this year, I tended to over treat to achieve this 'product' (a flat retina) and lost the perspective of the 'customer' (the patient's comfort, convenience and field of vision). Yes, more retinas were 'flat', (retinal surgeons are consumed by making a three-dimensional structure conform to a two-dimensional outcome!) but patients had more 'aggressive' surgery, more hospital visits, and perhaps less comfort and reduced peripheral vision. Note, only a 'flat retina' is required for our national audit standards again encouraging acceptable practice not excellence. At the end of this first year, I attended a conference and had a conversation over coffee with a senior London consultant I respected. He also recorded all his outcomes but, unlike me, had the IT skills to format the data into useful information! He commented on my wearing a belt and braces and a 'failure' conversation ensued! (I was not fearful of my trousers falling down. I liked braces but did not like the way they pulled my trousers up and out at the back, hence the belt. I digress!) As a result of this conversation, I realised that I had to embrace failure as fear of it was becoming ever constrictive and unhelpful. Trying to maintain perfection was high stress; it had become an obsession and was altering my approach to surgery. I had to learn to fail but to fail well and I have been on that journey ever since.

6.2   Surgical Failure—Adrenals, Heart and Head

Failure in surgery can be immediate and obvious to all present or, perhaps more often, immediate and hidden, only apparent to a trained observer or the surgeon. Regardless of observation or not, that feeling of your 'adrenals exploding' is unpleasant. Failure can occur within 48 h and require a 'return to theatre' (RTT), a metric that has to be reported as part of annual appraisal. That's a 'heart sink' moment when you thought all had gone well but alas, no! It is also an unpleasant feeling. Failure can also manifest months or years after the event making it almost impossible to connect directly to the original surgery and thus very difficult to learn from, more of a 'head scratch' moment and much less emotionally demanding. Success is much simpler and better all round although, reluctantly, I have to admit that failure is more likely to lead to improvement and progress (What doesn't kill you….). With failure, I fear for the patient's outcome. I feel a sense of shame and personal responsibility and that I am suddenly outside the group, a 'Tagged' zebra outside the herd suddenly visible to the local lions. I fear comparison and coming up short. It feels very isolating which may be significant in terms of my reactions to others failures in the current culture of surgery which I will discuss later. Failure has consequences, a bad outcome for my patient (although not always) and for me the threat of litigation and being struck off. Although I keep being told I am in a *no blame* culture and it is *the system* that has failed, much as I try, I don't believe it. My visceral response confirms this. I do not think I am alone in this although it has just occurred to me, I might be! Let's start our journey at the societal level.

6.3   Society Does Not Forget It—A Brief History of Failure

"There are these two young fish swimming along, and they happen to meet an older fish swimming the other way, who nods at them and says, "Morning, boys. How's the water?" And the two young fish swim on for a bit, and then eventually one of them looks over at the other and goes, "What the hell is water?"

David Foster Wallace (2005)

I will start in Ancient Greece where failure was viewed as something that could happen to anyone, 'good' or 'bad', it was not moralised. Fate was not determined by freewill. This understanding of failure suffused the culture with several notable plays reflecting and reinforcing it. The playwriter Sophocles wrote 'Oedipus the King' in 429 BC in Athens. It is a well-known Greek tragedy whereby Oedipus kills his father and marries his mother which I think you will agree ranks quite highly on the 'life significant failure' index. In spite of his failures the audiences were not left with the impression that *he* was a failure but rather that bad things do happen to good people and that kindness and sympathy should be shown to those who fail. When the Spartan army failed to defeat the Persian army at Thermopylae it was seen as a noble effort not a failure. Success and failure were simply a matter of circumstance.

The Roman Empire brought a very different approach to failure when it conquered Greece in 146 BC. Failure was no longer noble but shameful. Military triumph was celebrated, and competition was entertainment with gladiatorial contests and chariot racing common place. Winners and losers, success and failure, these were every day occurrences. To the losers, death and shame and to the winners, fame and fortune. Failure was now something to be anxious about. For example, in contrast to the Spartan experience of defeat, the Roman general Varus killed himself after losing a battle in the Tuetoburg forest. Failure was not noble but shameful. This is regarded by many as Rome's greatest defeat and the three legions that fought in the battle were disbanded and never fought again.

In a small occupied backwater within the Roman Empire, Jesus arrives and preaches that 'the first will be last', 'blessed are the meek' and that we have all fallen short, we are all sinners, we have all failed. 'Better to remove the plank from your own eye before attempting to remove the speck from your brother's eye' (sensible advice for an ophthalmologist) (*Matthew 7v5*). Christianity spread rapidly across Europe and subsequently the world forming the foundations of Western society (Holland 2019; Mangalwadi 2012). If we have *all* fallen short, if we have *all* failed, who are we to judge others when they fail? Accepting failure is actually a path to ultimate salvation.

In the East, Prince Siddhartha Gautama later known as the Buddha, realised that wealth and success could not bring humans satisfaction. Winning was not the answer, success can be found in apparent failure. He sought separation from the world of success to pursue a state where there is neither suffering, desire nor sense of self, Nirvana.

From the 1800s, the enlightenment era and the scientific revolution dominated Europe. Darwin put forward his 'Theory of Evolution' and the idea of 'survival of the fittest'. In this paradigm success meant life, failure extinction. In 1800, after the mass revolt against the privileged aristocracy, the French Revolution, Napoleon Bonaparte inaugurated a meritocracy. No longer did the minority enjoy success and wealth by virtue of birth, success was open to the talented not the privileged. However, failure was recategorised as not merely accidental nor morally neutral but, in some ways, deserved.

In the West, the 1980s brought a new idea of success. In 1987 Forbes published its first Rich list. Success was purely financial, and people could be measured, compared and ranked. This infamous decade perhaps had some of its roots in post-World War Two economic development when the nephew of Freud, Edward Bernays argued that production and consumption were key to financial prosperity in post-war America and subsequently Europe. The American dream saw great increases in the wealth of the middle classes over the 1950s and 1960s and little wealth inequality, the so called Great Compression. However, as the decades rolled on the dream was fast becoming a nightmare for many with soaring wealth inequality. The 1980s also brought us Neoliberal economics and deregulation of financial markets and the gap increased; everyone was a competitor now. This phase culminated (but did not end) with the global financial crisis in 2008. The Neoliberal economics of Alan Greenspan had made everyone a competitor in a game with winners and losers. Failure was significant once more, at least for the masses.

Our current cultural moment, with the ubiquitous internet and social media, has driven the consumer culture to new heights, now *we* are the products of digital capitalism. Social media provides almost constant comparison. We no longer try to 'Keep up with the Joneses', who presumably lived in the same street as us, now we are encouraged to keep up with everyone all the time and with their perfectly curated virtual lives. The result is anxiety, depression and increasing levels of suicide.

On reflection I think our current cultural moment, in the West at least, is perhaps the most intolerant of failure over the last 2000 years. In this post-Christian culture, the theology of original sin is gone and now we have not all fallen, some can be righteous and therefore others can be unrighteous. Judgement is now deserved and administered to all those on the wrong side of any issue. This polarisation is super-charged with social media and the internet. Failure is *identified*, even if this was in the past, *publicised* globally where comments can be made anonymously and without consequence, and then *immortalised* never to be forgotten. There is no forgiveness, no way back. I cannot think of a more toxic environment in which to fail. It feels like we have rapidly transitioned to an honour/shame culture, a blame culture and perhaps, even worse, a cancel culture.

In his book, 'Amusing ourselves to death', Neil Postman described three ages of society which have relevance to our current discussion and analysis (Postman 1985). In the first age, the 'oral age', societies passed down stories over generations and this was the norm up until the development of the printing press whereupon society entered the 'typographical age'. In this age words were written down and printed and distributed, they could be analysed and criticised and so great care was required in formulating ideas. He argued that this care and need for clarity and accuracy influenced speech in the culture at large. As a result, the entire culture was accustomed to debate and nuance with examples of political debates in town halls lasting many hours. His final age (the book was published in 1985) was assigned the 'televisual age' where presentation supplanted substance and every issue had to be dealt with quickly to fit in with the schedules. He argued that this change also influenced speech and thinking in the society at large. There was less substance-based discussion and nuance became difficult to explore, people became increasingly impatient. It is interesting to take his thinking and extrapolate it to the social media age we now find ourselves in where nuance has gone and even broad details are passed over with limits to Twitter currently 280 characters. Concentration is fleeting, headlines rule and polarisation is the norm. This further drives a lack of capability and capacity to even learn from failure because we find it difficult to pick apart the detail and nuance, it takes too much time. At the time of writing (2023) I am interested to see how the post-COVID investigation proceeds, can we learn anything? I certainly have less tolerance for reading complex articles and have a generalised impatience to solving complex problems compared to ten years ago.

Failure has never been more dangerous, more binary or more consequential. We no longer seem to care about the details or have the capacity to investigate and therefore might find it increasingly difficult to even learn from failure. Truth is relative in postmodernity. This is the water we swim in and it is within this water that healthcare and aviation sit. How does the aviation industry embrace failure and healthcare struggle with it? Can we really compare them and further, should we?

6.4 Healthcare and Aviation, Same Humans, Same Society but Different

"Learn from the mistakes of others, you can't live long enough to make them all yourself"
Eleanor Roosevelt

6.5 Failure Versus Scandal?

The airline industry responds positively to failure and is an ongoing source of comparison to the healthcare industry as we saw in 'Part I'. Should it be? In Aviation, failure sometimes means the loss of significant life including the pilots and crew involved. In healthcare, failure means loss of life or harm to the patient but not the medical staff involved. One could argue that it is in the pilots' interest to report *all* failures and near misses as their own lives may be at risk in future if they don't, although one day all surgeons will be patients! Major failure in aviation usually involves a single aircraft and is usually well publicised with the death of many people including the crew. Sympathy rather than moral outrage seems to be the response from society. Major failures in healthcare are rare but several come to mind and perhaps illustrate an intolerance to failure in healthcare not seen in aviation. The headlines rebadge these 'failures' as 'Scandals' such as the 'Bristol Heart Scandal', which we mentioned in 'Part I', blamed on the surgeons' learning curves. 'Failure' is defined as '*The fact of someone or something not succeeding*'; however, 'scandal' is defined as '*An action or event that causes a public feeling of shock and strong moral disapproval*'. The morality aspect of failure in healthcare is common. If any 'failure' could go public and be transformed into a 'scandal' does this encourage openness and honesty?

6.6   Data—Nowhere to Hide?

Aircraft have black boxes and cockpit voice recorders which deliver immense data to aid any investigation, none of which is admissible in court, further encouraging open disclosure. Failure is data rich and open to independent scrutiny. Aircraft deliver continuous data from the monitoring of each flight and this data is collected and analysed for patterns, even minor alterations in performance. Errors in healthcare are not data rich relying on self-reporting and eyewitness recollections from members of the medical team. Charts are available for review but unless surgery was performed through a digital visualising system able to record *and* being recorded at the time, *and* kept, little more detail is available. The closest we could get to aviation levels of data would be continuous video and audio recording of theatres and mandatory recording of all surgeries where possible (which also requires enhanced consent). I cannot see this happening in the current high pressured environment in the NHS although I am aware of specific hospitals outside the UK that do this and use the videos to assess complications with consequences for the surgeons who underperform at year end. Perhaps AI will solve these issues with constant monitoring and assessment of deviations from the standard although that is beginning to feel rather Orwellian and the resultant stress on surgeons might be detrimental to patient care as I discussed in 'Part I'. If we cannot eliminate human error, should we eliminate humans and move over to Robots? I do wonder how surgeons would respond to failure if it was clear that everyone would know about them anyway and if everyone knew about every failure, we might see that failure is perhaps more common than we thought. If we are all on the outside perhaps no one is?

6.7   No Blame Culture?

In aviation a 'no blame culture', where accidents are not stigmatised, facilitates investigation of the systems in place that resulted in the failure rather than the people involved. Near misses or minor errors can be reported with immunity if filed within 10 days of the incident. The Captain gave an example of a pilot missing a 'gate' on approach to Heathrow. The gate is an area in space through which the aircraft must pass and at a certain speed in order to proceed to landing. If the gate is missed, a 'go around' should be called. This 'go around' will automatically require a report to be filed by the crew and if there is anything unusual about the report there may be a call with the Fleet office. This conversation will go along the lines of 'well done on the go around' followed by 'why did this happen' and finally an encouragement that this 'will not happen again'. Although this 'no blame' culture has generally held true there are notable exceptions (NTSB 1978; Wilkinson 1993). One of my patients, who was a Captain, flew into Heathrow immediately after one of the most infamous near misses in UK aviation history, the November Oscar incident. The pilot involved, William Glen Stewart, was put on trial, charged, lost his license and subsequently took his own life. The headline seemed clear and that he was to blame but the details showed multiple contributing and mitigating factors. In healthcare we often talk about the 'Swiss Cheese model', there are times when all the holes just line up. Healthcare is attempting a 'no blame culture' but it is struggling.

Even in our local Morbidity and Mortality meetings, designed to highlight failures and near misses so we can all learn, blame does not seem far from the surface. In one incident a consultant apologised that a doctor's name had appeared on a slide detailing a complication. If we truly believed it is about systems not individuals this would not matter but it clearly does. When I have a complication, I certainly blame myself and, in the moment, cannot see the 'system' or 'process' that has let me down. However, I need to blame myself in order to learn and get better, I have a high Internal LOC. Surgeons tend to exhibit high trait conscientiousness on the 5 Factor model of personality which I will explore further in 'Part III'. This is likely to lead to higher levels of self-criticism and I would argue might subtly influence the culture within medicine perpetuating a negative spiral when it comes to embracing failure. If we blame ourselves, we are likely to apply the same standards to other's errors and blame them. For example, this is my honest reaction to someone else's failure in a typical corridor conversation. On hearing the news there is an immediate response and it is a positive emotion. I would not go as far as to say pleasure or schadenfreude but more a relief that comes from knowing someone else is fallible, they are on the outside and you are on the inside safe from harm *on this occasion*. Following this reaction there is a need to understand what went wrong. Because I have very high standards and blame myself for everything it is natural for me to apply the same high standards to the surgeon in question. If we add in the 'false attribution error' which we will cover in 'Part III' we have the perfect scenario for criticism of the surgeon. However, after the judgement comes the realisation that I have made the same errors and many more. The end emotion is sympathy and a sense of 'There but for the grace of God go I'. Perhaps I am outside the normal range of surgeons but if surgeons do mirror this response curve, we might be able to challenge the culture and skip the first two stages and realise we are all fallible. Pilots truly believe they are fallible, surgeons do not.

I discussed the blame culture with The Captain and asked him about his corridor conversations following errors as these often get to the heart of the true culture. His response was that following identification of the pilot there would be an immediate, 'That could have been me, I need to understand what happened'. I tried to push him on any value judgement that might arise even in the millisecond between identification of the pilot and the error but it is clear, all pilots believe they are fallible. I also spoke to a GP and an anaesthetist and although these in no way provide evidence of a blame/no blame culture in their respective fields the responses were similar. The anaesthetist admitted that several years ago there may have been an element of judgement and criticism however, in recent years he felt all anaesthetists would respond in a similar manner, that the error could have been them and they are all keen to learn. The GP, who investigates medical errors, said that rather than judge the doctor the first thought was, given the circumstances, it could have been him. What is it with surgeons?

It seems we blame ourselves, other surgeons and, increasingly, patients want to blame us given the rise in litigation costs in the NHS. In a survey by the Medical Defence Union, 30% of doctors feared being blamed or facing legal action for making mistakes (Richardson 2022). In the NHS, clinical negligence claims in England rose from £582 million in 2006 to 2007 to £2.2 billion in 2020 to 2021. I am struggling with a no blame culture, it's everywhere!

6.8 Reporting Failure

The GMC guidelines on the 'Duty of Candour' state

> Every health and care professional must be open and honest with patients and people in their care when something that goes wrong with their treatment or care causes, or has the potential to cause, harm or distress.

This feels quite a nebulous request. What constitutes 'going wrong', what is 'harm' and what is 'potential' and how do we define 'distress'. For example, in cataract surgery the opening in the capsular bag, the capsulorrhexis, should ideally be round and just smaller than the optic of the lens. If it is very small the patient may develop phimosis (scarring and contraction) of the capsule and a risk of zonule weakness and late dislocation of the lens many years later. If it is too large there is a risk of refractive instability and even the lens dislocating from within the bag. When is it *too* small or *too* large? Reporting not only relies on honesty but also a threshold for what that doctor feels triggers the need for candour and that might depend on their own standards of care. The airline industry is far more prescriptive with multiple SOPs dictating behaviour, deviation is more easily detected.

As I have discussed, there are some well-defined and specific complications at the procedural level that have to be reported for appraisal and audit by each surgeon. These are very few in number compared to all the possible complications and often have no actual effect on the outcome for the patient. At a level above there are 'Serious Untoward Incidents' (SUIs) and 'Never Events' that have to be reported and investigated and form part of any assessment of the institution by the Care Quality Commission (CQC). A SUI is 'an event that occurs which has caused or has the potential to cause, serious harm to the patient and requires a formal investigation'. Never Events are 'serious, largely preventable safety incidents that should not occur if the available safety measures are implemented'. Both are rare in comparison to the number of procedural complications at the level below and perhaps act as 'Canaries in the coal mine', a reflection or indication of the general safety culture. One common Never Event in Ophthalmology is the insertion of the wrong intraocular lens. The wrong lens is not defined as a suboptimal outcome (of great importance to the patient), but simply a deviation from the plan even if the plan was, on reflection, suboptimal. This Never Event is reasonably straightforward to deal with and may not need any remedial action if the patient is happy and can see well. It is significant for the institution but not always for the patient.

6.9   Learning from Failure—Sharing and Relevance

In aviation, the failure reports are available to everyone in the industry and all the airlines have a responsibility to implement the findings. The Captain gets a regular bulletin that every pilot has to read and sign to say they have read. One failure will result in learnings that are very widespread throughout the industry, even globally. In healthcare there are national alerts, 'Field Safety notices' published in response to alerts from manufacturers regarding medical devices and medicines but with health-care, such a vast and diverse discipline, most of these notices are irrelevant to most doctors most of the time. Hospitals employ internal IT systems designed to capture complications and near misses and have to report 'SUIs' and 'Never Events' as well as a range of common complications to benchmark surgeons. All these require reporting by staff as they are not automatically captured and rely on all staff to subse-quently read the report findings. Investigations rely on teams gathered from among the existing (busy) staff to investigate and generate the report. Morbidity and Mortality meetings are held regularly within specific departments to try to aid shared learning but it seems difficult to learn the lessons even within specific departments let alone specific hospitals, let alone nationally or globally as in the airline industry. In my experience of these meetings, failure generally results in additional measures being added to the existing processes like the snowball I discussed previously with regard to lean surgery. There is a real danger of a 'tick box' culture resulting in reduced volume, reduced efficiency and, ironically, less safety. There are examples of Hospi-tals embracing failure and benefitting significantly in terms of reduced complications and reduction in litigation as exampled by the Virginia Mason Hospital in Seattle where there was 74% reduction in insurance premiums due to reduced litigation following the introduction of a reporting system for errors and near misses (Syed 2015). This particular culture changed following a traumatic incident with a patient that forced disparate teams to come together. Jeremy Hunt invited members from the Virginia Mason Institute to 5 Trusts in the UK in 2015 with some positive results but I am not aware of any national guidance that has resulted from their visit.

The current levels of safety in aviation are the direct result of learnings from many fatal and non-fatal accidents and near misses. Several fatal incidents have led to marked improvements in safety over the years both in terms of interactions among the crew and even giving birth to the discipline of ergonomics in the cockpit. Significant advances in medicine have also come about as a result failure in well-designed clinical trials. In these trials failure is built in as comparisons of interventions are made. Healthcare research embraces failure and has made huge progress, clinical medicine perhaps less so. Failure is critical for the learning surgeon as they try to develop new skills and techniques. I use 'learning' and not 'trainee' because all surgeons need to be able to learn new techniques throughout their careers.

6.10 The Spectrum of Failure—Surgeon to System

As I think through my own complications, I realise they actually occur at multiple levels along a spectrum hence I often struggle to see how 'the System' has failed as it always seems to be my fault. If we imagine a spectrum of influences, at one end the surgeon's hands and their circle of 'control' at the other end the System and culture at large. In the middle we move from aspects the surgeon can directly influence through to surgical teams and equipment. Failure is a mix of factors; we might blame ourselves but fail to take into account the system or blame the system and fail to take into account our own responsibility. It's not binary.

Furthest from 'the system', are the individual steps of surgical technique. These may not be performed perfectly according to my 'Lean' approach to surgery guided by 'goal setting theory' in terms of the 'mini-games' I aspire to play perfectly. No harm is done to the patient in failure, it's just not perfect. I can learn from this level and improve and further, failure does not hurt my identity and does not affect the patient outcome. Surgeons will also differ in terms of what constitutes 'perfection' in each step and may not even attend to 'micro-technique' in the first place. Failure here is common and critical to improvement and simulators offer great advantages, up to a point, at this level. The surgeon is mostly responsible at this level.

Failures slightly closer to 'the system' can be found at the procedural level. At this level there will be defined complications that are used as part of annual appraisal with set standards required to be met by the surgeon which I have already argued in 'Part I', encourage adequate care rather than excellent care. Unlike at the micro-technique level, many complications at the procedural level are unusual or unique and even with reviewing video footage are difficult to learn from. They do not necessarily result in a poor outcome for the patient. To learn from failure at this level requires me to review surgery and apply 'System 2' thinking which I will cover in 'Part III'. The system may have more reach into this area than the micro-technique level. For example, the system may influence failure if I am required to do too many cases due to waiting list pressure or if I am required to participate in multiple activities in theatre beyond the actual responsibility of delivering surgery which can cause me to become distracted. I have seen my additional responsibilities increase dramatically over the years.

Moving further along the spectrum, team dynamics, performance and human factors can play a critical role in failure. It is in this region I think many surgeons underestimate the effect of non-technical skills (NTS) on complications rates. NTS include cognitive and interpersonal skills, communication, leadership, situational awareness and decision-making. In one study, deficits in human factors and communication were identified as a root cause in over 60% of all the sentinel events reviewed by the Joint Commission between 2004 and 2013 (The Joint Commission 2013). A sentinel even is defined as a patient safety event that results in death, permanent harm or severe temporary harm. Poor teamwork can result in increased complication rates and poorer outcomes for patients (Mazzocco et al. 2009). In another study, 43% of errors were attributed to poor communication (Gawande et al. 2003). I have certainly experienced increased stress as a result of teams that are not familiar with the procedures or not trained in the specifics of my subspecialty. In this situation, I find I need to concentrate well beyond the surgical field and this is difficult and distracting like driving and trying to read a map at the same time (yes, we used to have to do this once). Working with a well-trained team, especially a scrub nurse who knows you well, is truly magnificent and surgery flows. The debrief at the end of surgery is useful for identifying issues at this level. Healthcare has learned lessons from aviation in this area but also from Formula 1 with Williams engaging the neonatal team at the University Hospital of Wales (UHW) in Cardiff to improve teamwork and efficiency on the neonatal unit (Williams 2016).

Moving further along the spectrum we approach the 'system'. The system has significant influence over work schedules and planning of theatres, policies, staff training and development and the general culture, in terms of safety and bureaucracy, which is heavily influenced by societal culture at large. Being overworked has been a common source of error in surgery, up to 33% in one paper (Gawande et al. 2003). The 'safety culture' mentioned previously can also interfere with the surgery. Where I personally find the system unhelpful is in the demands put upon me beyond the actual surgery. I have worked in various environments and have experienced the effect these can have on the flow of surgery, efficiency and outcomes. In the NHS I have experienced a general additive approach to safety resulting in cumbersome and burdensome protocols and a requirement for me to do multiple tasks in addition to doing the surgery often in the pursuit of safety. The most efficient and often safest units ensure the surgeon focusses on surgery and nothing else. The Aravind Hospital in India is a good example. Here we see an even lighter touch in terms of safety and bureaucracy but excellent volumes and outcomes, often exceeding our results in the West, and lower infection rates (Chang 2019; Templeton 2023). Anchoring is a very powerful heuristic, which I will discuss in 'Part III' that can normalise and tether approaches to surgery. I will show you a Japanese Surgeon who puts our high-volume surgery to shame.

6.11   Avoiding Failure

Failure in surgery is inevitable. If we try too hard to protect the trainees (and therefore patients) from failure we can interfere with the quality and completeness of training resulting in consultants who do not feel confident to deal with common complications. I only felt I transitioned from 'technician' to 'surgeon' when I dealt with my own complications. For example, the most common audit standard used in ophthalmology is the rate of posterior capsular rupture (PCR) in cataract surgery. PCR does not necessarily result in a poor outcome for the patient but is easy to identify. In a study I completed with a trainee we found nearly 80% of trainees lacked confidence to deal with PCR without senior support as a result of lack of experience in dealing with it (Turnbull and Lash 2016).

6.12   Summary

Perhaps I cannot see *'the system'* in my failures because most of my failures occur at the surgical end of the continuum rather than the system end and it is easy not to notice the subtle influences at this micro-level like culture, bureaucracy, work load and division of labour in theatre. It is no good trying to persuade me that failures are failures of the system and I should feel comfortable reporting them because my visceral response tells me otherwise. I should feel more comfortable reporting them because we all have failures and the culture needs to shift so that we all truly believe this.

6.13   The Culture of Surgery and Its Influence on Failure

6.13.1   Introduction

I have touched briefly on culture in terms of a 'no blame' culture; but in this section, I want to go deeper into culture and how it might facilitate or hinder a 'no blame' culture. In writing this section I am relying on my personal experiences of several hospitals I have worked in within the UK NHS system and a public hospital in Australia. My experience is therefore limited to a small sample of hospitals and the culture may well be very different in other units. My experience of culture is limited to my speciality and I am aware that not all medical specialties will have the same culture, even other surgical specialities. I also view these cultures through my own personality. I have attempted to understand the culture within the airline industry by interviewing The Captain. Again, I am aware that this is one pilot's observations and experience within a specific company and airlines certainly differ in terms of the corporate environment. In this way I may well be missing aspects of culture outside these limited perspectives but my hope for this section is to give you lenses which will allow you to view and reflect on your own culture and how it regards failure.

6.14   Goffee and Jones

I will explore organisational culture based on the model proposed by Goffee and Jones (Goffee 1996). Clearly there are multiple other perspectives, but I find this particular model useful. It assesses culture through a sociological lens on two dimensions, Sociability and Solidarity and at two levels, high or low. This reveals four cultures, Networked, Mercenary, Communal and Fragmented (Fig. 6.2).

From 'What Holds the modern Company together?' by Goffee, R and Jones, G November–December 1996.Copyright ©1996 by Harvard Business Publishing; all rights reserved.

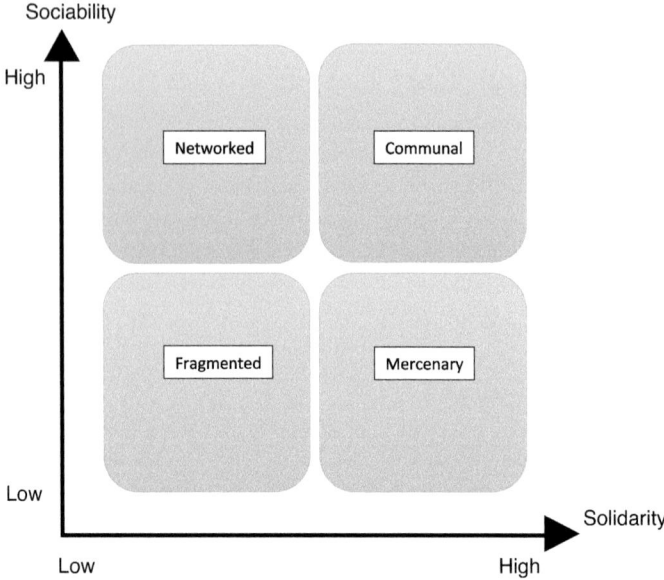

Fig. 6.2 Two Dimensions, Four cultures (Goffee and Jones 1996)

Sociability is a measure of sincere friendliness among members of the organisation. Solidarity is a measure of the ability of the group to pursue shared objectives effectively regardless of personal ties. Highly sociable environments are characterised by sincere friendships where people will work harder to help each other out and will often go the extra mile. Think of a not-for-profit start-up company doing something everyone is passionate about. Although perhaps highly enjoyable to work in, the downside of these cultures is they can suffer from tolerating poor performance as there is often an exaggerated concern for consensus and avoiding conflict. Failure might be ignored. If sociability resides in the heart, then solidarity resides in the head. In an environment high in solidarity, relationships are formed in the pursuit of a common goal and poor performance is not tolerated; the goal is paramount. Trade unions are a classic example of high solidarity cultures but Goffee and Jones also suggest that doctors and lawyers, not known for high levels of solidarity, can exhibit high solidarity when an external threat is manifest. Perhaps think of the Virginia Mason Hospital turnaround. Solidarity can come and go however sociability is more permanent. It is also important to note that in larger organisations different cultures can manifest at different levels and this is especially true for NHS Hospitals. Different cultures may be seen between departments and specialities and even between subspecialities. Perhaps take some time to reflect on your own immediate culture on these two dimensions.

I currently work in the NHS in the UK and do some private work in a specialty that has a vibrant private sector, Ophthalmology. This will influence the culture and so its limitations must be noted and not generalised. However, I have generally experienced a low sociability and low solidarity culture among surgeons, a 'Fragmented' culture. I have been thinking through the reasons for this although I may be guilty of the 'Crime of Procrustes' in exploring it. Am I simply seeing what I am looking for and making it fit?

Entry in to surgical training is highly competitive with competition ratios up to 1 in 53 in some specialities in the UK (NHS Health and education England 2022). Failure is common in the highly competitive post-graduate examinations where only 30% of the doctors actually pass certain exams, the rest having to re-sit, often several times, with some having to leave their chosen speciality and retrain. Failure has significant consequences on career progression. Might this explain the low solidarity given that surgeons are in competition with each other? Sociability is not helped by the constant competition and the challenges of balancing a very busy work life with study and a personal life. The low solidarity and low sociability put the culture in the fragmented box. In a fragmented culture the members often believe they work for themselves. If asked what I do at a party I usually respond 'I am an Eye Surgeon' rather than 'I work at University Hospital Southampton. In a fragmented culture there can be negative corridor conversations as members try to sabotage others especially where there is a significant element of competitive practice availability or research prowess at stake. One person's failure might be another's gain. In a fragmented culture sociability is also low, there is little to no socialisation outside work. I have organised several Christmas parties and found it very difficult to get all the consultants out for the night! However, the nurses' coffee rooms are adorned with various 'group selfies' taken at parties indicating high sociability and they can often be seen visiting colleagues when on annual leave! However, Goffee and Jones suggest that this 'Fragmented' culture can work well in professional organisations with highly trained individuals working in very different areas. This seems very appropriate for healthcare in the UK which is increasingly super specialist. In the NHS each subspecialty tends to attract different types of people with each having specific specialist knowledge not known by others and each with its own unique set of problem and issues to face as individual business units. There is little transfer of care between subspecialities.

Have another look at Fig. 6.2 and think through your own immediate environment. Although formal assessment is available, just thinking it through can be helpful. Do you agree that a fragmented culture seems to be the worst culture in which to fail? I would also suggest that a communal culture, high in both sociability and solidarity, might be the most conducive to embracing failure but perhaps, not learning from it?

6.15 Airline Industry Culture

To try to understand the culture let us return to the career path of the pilot. I discussed this briefly in Chap. 2 with The Captain and it is useful to keep the surgical career path in the background to compare and contrast the two professions. Getting a commercial pilot's licence is not competitive. You need around £150 K. Once you have a licence there is significant competition for jobs, especially among certain global airlines. It may be the pilot gets their first job in a more local airline and then looks to move across with more experience. The other route is to be granted a sponsorship deal with an airline. They will pay for the commercial pilot's licence and then, provided the pilot performs and is competent, they may be offered a position. Competition for sponsorship is very significant. However, once the pilot is employed, progression is based on seniority. Provided you stay with the same airline you will eventually be offered a captain's post and provided you pass the required competences you will be given the job. If you change airlines you will return to the bottom rung and earn seniority year by year. In this sense there is no competition between pilots in post, everyone knows who is next to be offered promotion. Additionally, there is no 'private' work for airline pilots and senior pilots are looked after very well with excellent salaries and retirement provision. In surgery competition is fierce at every stage and private work provides further competition until retirement.

Given the career path for pilots, I would expect lower levels of competition and therefore higher levels of solidarity among pilots. Unions are active in the airline industry which reinforces and signals this high solidarity. I asked The Captain what he thought and he recounted his experiences over the various crises that have hit the airline industry during his time including oil shocks, economic collapses, wars, terrorist attacks and finally COVID. Following the September 11th terrorist attack a large meeting was organised for all the pilots. One very senior captain spoke up and suggested that 'they were not going to lose any pilots', to which another, less senior, captain responded in protest but was quickly put in his place. They did not lose any pilots; they all took a pay cut. This is incredible solidarity, a sense that they were all in it together. It was only during COVID that some pilots were released perhaps because the pain had to be shared at all levels in this exceptional period. In terms of sociability, they do not often meet in person but there was a sense, from talking with The Captain, that there is a high level of comradery and socialisation occurs through virtual means and infrequent person to person contact. This would put the culture into the 'communal' sector which I would argue is the best culture to fail in although failure might be tolerated too much. Going back to the corridor conversation in the previous section on failure, there is a core belief that all pilots are fallible and that the initial response to hearing of a failure was to learn from it. In this way failure has a high value and will not be ignored, nor will the pilot who failed be punished or suffer reputational damage, they all believe (really believe) they are fallible.

6.16   The Visceral Clash of Cultures—Airline Versus Surgery

During a separate interview with The Captain on 'approaches to problem solving', the stark visceral reality of our culture crash manifested quite unexpectedly. We were exploring the problem that becomes apparent during the flight, not a predictable event identified at one of the pre-flight briefs and not a 'Mayday' situation. The Captain gave an example of flying into Dalaman airport. Every runway at every airport has mandated visibility requirements in order to proceed to a landing and at Dalaman this is a minimum cloud base of 720 feet and visibility of 2.4 km which equates to becoming visual with the runway at approximately 2.5 (nautical) miles (talk about mixing units!). Landing begins with the descent from the cruising altitude around 37,000 feet, down to 4300 feet which represents the approach platform from which the final critical part of the approach and landing commences. Provided the criteria are met it is perfectly acceptable and legal to proceed to land. This represents a hard stop, a bottom line a SOP. However, we discussed what might happen if mid-flight, at the approach brief, weather reports suggested that thunder storms were moving in on Dalaman, cloud base was dropping and visibility was deteriorating. We now have a possible deviation from the requirements as weather changes, so how does The Captain decide what to do and when? The Captain and first officer would 'notice' the change, 'understand' the consequences and 'think ahead', another useful framework pilots use. Note problem solving is a joint affair. At this point our discussion began to feel very much like a discussion I would have with a fellow surgeon discussing how they might manage a potential deviation from the usual and it proved equally hard to extract what would actually be done as we sat drinking coffee, trying to pretend we were actually in the aircraft and decisions actually had to be made! That is because there are many influences on any decision which are constantly in flux. The Captain suggested that every pilot had their own 'bottom line'. I was interested if experience determined this, after all I know that experienced surgeons would take on more risky cases. In other words, was there wriggle room in the decision-making process up to and prior to the mandatory hard stop at the final decision point (2.5 miles)? After much discussion, and bearing in mind I am not a pilot, I was very much in favour of not trying to land if the current status was not at the required limits, before the final descent, saving fuel to go onto the next airport. However, The Captain suggested that most of the time the pilot will approach intending to land aborting only at the last decision point quite appropriately and legally. I suggested, quite honestly and with my guard down in full surgical mode, that if the pilot had made a decision that was far closer to the bottom line than another pilot and an incident occurred, it would be the pilot's 'fault'. The Captain looked at me somewhat taken aback and said it would be described as a 'poor decision'. I could not help myself as a surgeon. There was wriggle room with a degree of autonomy to make a poor decision and therefore 'fault' surely was a possibility. Surgically, I have been in situations just like this where a case is suboptimal in terms of view or tissue responses but I have ploughed on, almost using muscle memory, completing the case safely where as I know that as a trainee I would have stopped and let the boss take over. I have dealt with cases from experienced colleagues who have got into trouble and I have referred cases onto others when it has happened to me. Temperament, experience and competence all come into play and error might result. However, if I continue a suboptimal case and get a complication perhaps it really was a poor decision to continue rather than my 'fault' I had the complication. Could surgeons believe this? That would certainly help our culture in terms of embracing failure and learning from it!

6.17 Medical/Aviation Culture Conclusion

If I am correct the two industries represent very different cultures and by chance, I would argue, appear to be at opposite ends of the spectrum in terms of facilitating a 'No blame' culture. The low solidarity, low sociability 'Fragmented' culture in surgery seems the least likely to embrace a 'No blame' culture out of the four, whereas the high solidarity, high sociability 'Communal' culture might just be the most likely to embrace it. There is no competition in the airline industry beyond entrance and pilots are well looked after with seniority. Surgeons compete to get in, compete to get up and for many, compete to get out into the world of business and research with personal and professional reputation their key currency.

6.18 The Self

In this final section I will look at the perception of 'The Self' and how this has evolved over time. I am interested in how 'The Self' influences our perception of failure. Is it failure of what we do, or increasingly who we are? I am mindful that once again I am paddling in the shallows of the oceans of knowledge out there. I have a new respect for Philosophy and its subtle and incredibly powerful effects on society but it is way beyond the scope of this book, and my knowledge, to go swimming in the deep. I will keep my feet on the sands in the shallows! For those interested I found two books of great help (Storr 2017; Trueman 2020).

The western idea of self was born in Ancient Greece. With little land to farm on and multiple islands to fish off, it was a very atomised society. The ideal physical form was demonstrated by art and the statues of the gods. Think of Atlas and Adonis. Academic prowess was highly respected, think of Plato and Aristotle. Individual athletic performance was celebrated, think of the Olympics. The stories told in Ancient Greece were the classical hero arcs still seen in most current movie plots. The hero has humble beginnings, is faced with a quest, rises to the challenge, fails temporarily but then overcomes and in the end wins. However, in the East the Confucian concept of the self was firmly nestled in family and society with the stories told more ambiguous, more complex and more societal. Failure was experienced when letting these people down rather than personal failure. I will focus on the Western self but it is important to realise that the concept of the self, even today, appears different between different cultures, we just get used to the water we swim in.

In the West the modern self has rapidly moved to the centre of culture and is almost beyond challenge supported by increasing legislation and driven by social media. The atomised self in the West started in Ancient Greece but thinkers over the last 200 years have tilled the soil that is enabling the current view of self to flourish and atomisation has returned. They include, among others, Rousseau, Nietzsche, Freud, Rogers, Reiff, Marx, Foucault and Sartres. I cannot begin to explore this topic, it is vast. I want to focus on one element of the self that came out of the 1980s and I think heavily influences our approach to failure, Self-Esteem.

6.19 Self-esteem

The self-esteem movement exploded out of the political scene in California in 1989 following publication of the 'Social importance of Self-Esteem' published by the 'California Task Force to Promote Self-Esteem and Personal and Social Responsibility' led by John Vasconcellos (Mecca 1989). John believed that Self-Esteem could be the vaccine against most societal ills from crime and drugs to pollution. It spread into schools across America and then into Europe. It spread into organisations and influenced CEOs. After several years of almost unchallenged influence research began to find issues with the science. David Shannahoff-Khalsa, part of the original 'California Task Force' refused to sign the final publication with major concerns over its authenticity and exaggeration of the links found by the academics on the working group (Storr 2017). Among others, Baumeister challenged the assumption that high self-esteem could cause the many positive outcomes as claimed (Baumeister et al. 2003).

Not only were the claims made found to be false, the millennials educated under this new philosophy subsequently showed an increase in narcissism year on year. Jean Twenge thought that the self-esteem movement was at least one factor in explaining why millennials had higher self-esteem and were more likely to see themselves as above average than previous generations and why they scored higher on measures of narcissistic personality traits (Twenge 2014). The self-esteem movement focussed attention on the self as a positive entity and encouraged praise for minimal achievement especially in schools. In spite of fundamental flaws in the original work and ongoing challenges to the concept, self-esteem is alive and well today. Failure does not sit well in this hyper positive, hyper affirming environment where no one is actually allowed to fail. Has this movement conflated in our minds what we do with who we are?

6.20 Culture—Conclusion

Society seems to tolerate failure less each year. I am not sure there is anything we can do except be aware of it and challenge it where we can, if we are brave enough.

At the industry level I compared and contrasted medicine and aviation. The airline industry has embraced failure but does tend to have a data rich environment which in itself might encourage disclosure of errors or near misses as there is nowhere to hide! Aviation has an open attitude to failure and responds quickly, and generally impersonally, to each failure with a couple of notable and tragic exceptions. From my conversation with The Captain, it seems a 'Communal' culture is most likely and this is perhaps the best culture in which to fail. I am convinced all pilots believe they are truly fallible, even in corridor conversations, and this is critical in embracing failure. Medicine is less data rich and much more diverse making understanding and sharing failure more difficult. The competitive nature of surgery does not encourage openness and surgeons tend towards a high internal LOC. As a result, surgeons tend to be hard on themselves and others as reflected by the typical corridor conversations I have heard. The culture is perhaps best described as a 'Fragmented' culture, perhaps the worst culture in which to fail. However, in surgery there is a spectrum of influence on failure from the surgeon's own hands to the system and culture at large. Each end influences failure to varying degrees and it is rarely all the Surgeon's fault or all the system's fault. Unless we can change the culture such that we surgeons really do believe we are fallible *as a first response* change will be difficult.

At the core of my 'failure nest,' is our identity. Who we are seems so much entangled with what we do and is driven by a sense that we are all special in the Self-Esteem sense. Perhaps failure as a surgeon is to fail at who you are not what you do. It is a question worth asking yourself and if you don't, retirement might be a shock.

Although fear of failure is perhaps a barrier to 'Lean' surgery, 'Lean surgery' and 'Goal setting theory' might also provide the opportunity for embracing failure and learning from it especially at the micro-technique level. Failure is inevitable and, rather than avoiding it, we need to truly accept it and learn to fail well but also not to fail to learn well.

6.21 To Try

How is failure portrayed in your local media?

Reflect on a failure and analyse the contributing factors from your hands to the system.

How did you feel about this failure? What did it say about you?

How much was under your control or influence?

Reflect on your local culture—which quadrant might you be in and how will that influence attitudes to failure?

References

Baumeister RF, Campbell JD, Krueger JI, Vohs KD. Does high self-esteem cause better performance, interpersonal success, happiness, or healthier lifestyles? Psychol Sci the Public Interest. 2003;4(1):1–44. https://doi.org/10.1111/1529-1006.01431.

Chang D (2019) Lesson from the world's greatest team of cataract surgeons. Cataract Surgery: Telling It Like It Is.

Gawande AA, Zinner MJ, Studdert DM, Brennan TA. Analysis of errors reported by surgeons at three teaching hospitals. Surgery. 2003;133(6):614–21. https://doi.org/10.1067/msy.2003.169.

Goffee RJG. What holds the modern company together. Harvard Business Revie 1996.

Holland T. Dominion: the making of the western mind. Little, Brown; 2019.

Mangalwadi, V. The book that made your world: How the bible created the soul of the western civilisation; 2012.

Mazzocco K, Petitti DB, Fong KT, Bonacum D, Brookey J, Graham S, Lasky RE, Sexton JB, Thomas EJ. Surgical team behaviors and patient outcomes. Am J Surg. 2009;197(5):678–85. https://doi.org/10.1016/j.amjsurg.2008.03.002.

Mecca A, SNJ, VJ. (1989) The social importance of self esteem.

NHS Health and education England. *Competition ratios for 2022*. https://Medical.Hee.Nhs.Uk/Medical-Training-Recruitment/Medical-Specialty-Training/Competition-Ratios/2022-Competition-Ratios

NTSB. https://www.ntsb.gov/investigations/AccidentReports/Reports/AAR7907.pdf. NTSB; 1978.

Postman N. Amusing ourselves to death: Public discourse in the age of show business. Penguin; 1985.

Richardson, J. 3 in 10 doctors fear being blamed or facing legal action after admitting mistakes. GP Online; 2022.

Storr W. Selfie: how we became so Self-obsessed and what its doing to us. Picador; 2017.

Syed M. Black box thinking. Portfolio/Penguin; 2015.

Templeton, S. Fear of a microbial planet: how safety culture makes us less safe. Brownstone Institute; 2023.

The Joint Commision. Sentinel event data: root causes by event type (2004-June 2013); 2013. https://www.Medleague.Com/Wp-Content/Uploads/2013/11/Root_Causes_by_Event_Type_2004-2Q2013.Pdf.

Trueman CR. The rise and triumph of the modern self: cultural amnesia. Crossway: Expressive Individualism and the road to Sexual Revolution; 2020.

Turnbull AMJ, Lash SC. Confidence of ophthalmology specialist trainees in the management of posterior capsule rupture and vitreous loss. Eye. 2016;30(7):943–8. https://doi.org/10.1038/eye.2016.55.

Twenge JM. Generation me: why today's young Americans are more confident, assertive. Entitled And more Miserable than Ever Before: Atria Books; 2014.

Wilkinson S. Text of article commissioned by "Air and Space Smithsonian" magazine, Autumn 1993. "The November Oscar Incident." 1993. http://Picma.Info/Sites/Default/Files/Documents/Events/November%20Oscar%20article.Pdf.

Williams. 2016. Williams pit stop expertise to help save newborn babies.

Part III
The 'Why' of Surgery

Introduction

In 'Part I', I explored surgery as experienced in the 'surgical field' in the moment of surgery, the 'how' of surgery. In 'Part II', I explored surgery 'around the head' of the surgeon in terms of planning and specifically the application of 'Lean' principles and the barriers to this approach especially in term of failure, the 'what' of surgery. In 'Part III', I will move into the 'air the surgeon breathes' in theatre and beyond, the 'why' of surgery. I will delve into the assumptions we all have about how the world works and how these assumptions influence the other boxes downstream. This box is like the tiny rudder on a large ship hidden beneath the waves but ultimately determining direction.

I will demonstrate how in life generally, and in surgery specifically, we prefer to function on automatic pilot by exploring 'System 1' and 'System 2' thinking. I will discuss how experts and novices differ in solving complex problems and how the trainee needs to develop schemas, not just technique, to progress surgically and how simulators might actually interfere with this process. Automatic pilot generally works well until it doesn't. We need to ensure Procrustes does not get hold of Occam's razor.

I will then review common Heuristics as applied to surgery and how they might interfere with our intention to become better surgeons. There is significant overlap with 'lean' surgery in terms of eliminating 'Muda' and embracing 'Kaizen' from 'Part II' and sports psychology and goal setting theory from 'Part I'. I will also explore their effects on clinical audit and suggest the need for a more nuanced approach to this professionally required activity.

Finally, I will look at personality through the lenses of the Myers Briggs type indicator (MBTI) and the Big Five Factor Model of Personality. What effect does personality have on the practice of surgery, if any, and is there a surgical personality? I am grateful to all of my previous Fellows but especially those who completed both these personality assessments to help me explore the role of personality in surgery and, in the spirit of full disclosure, I will reveal my own results. I am hoping to tie personality with surgical behaviour so I can train Fellows in a bespoke fashion, but let's see if this is the case. Once more I apologise for paddling in the shallows, there is another ocean of knowledge out there in this arena.

Chapter 7
Problem Solving—What Can We Learn from Grand Chess Masters and Speed Cubers?

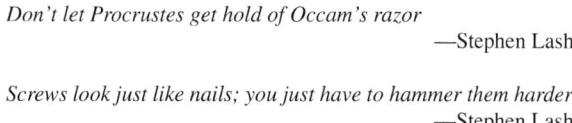

Don't let Procrustes get hold of Occam's razor
—Stephen Lash

Screws look just like nails; you just have to hammer them harder
—Stephen Lash

Abstract You are an experienced surgeon faced with a difficult case, a complex reoperation for example. You look and almost immediately have a plan of action and execute it effortlessly. Your trainee asks you afterwards why you did what you did and it actually takes effort to dissect your thinking but they are clearly impressed. During the discussion you wonder if certain aspects of the surgery might have been better another way but don't let on, why ruin a perfectly good moment? You continue to think about this later that evening whilst reading a bedtime story to your child and feel rather guilty about not giving them your full attention. Actually, you can't remember reading anything at all, but you do have a plan for doing the surgery differently next time!

Keywords System 1 thinking · System 2 thinking · Automatic pilot · Cognitive load theory (CLT) · Surgeon's performance · Surgical decision-making · Surgery improvement · Patient outcome

7.1 System 1 and System 2 Thinking

In 'Part II' I argued how changes in western culture may have shifted the population from being intellectually rigorous and informed, through a population influenced more by appearance and presentation over content to arrive at our current 'Social media age' where headlines rule and details are optional. Nuance is dead and this may form an important barrier to learning if we are not careful. We have talked about 'failing well' but we also need to 'learn well' from those failures. Learning takes time and effort but we increasingly prefer 'life hacks' and 'magic' as opposed to slow, deliberate 'formation'. In his book 'Thinking Fast and Slow', Daniel Kahneman explored what he called System 1 and System 2 thinking (Kahneman 2011). These are not explanations of how the brain works but rather useful observations and should be seen as caricatures that facilitate understanding.

System 1 is the automatic system which is very fast and in constant operation. It is so fast that we will act on its instruction before we have realised what is going on. Pulling your hand away from a hot plate that you just grasped or grimacing at vomit on the floor. It is active when you are chatting to a friend whilst driving and even during routine, uncomplicated surgery. It is also active when reading a simple story to your child, whilst thinking about your surgery earlier that day, and arriving at the last page with no recollection of reading anything! It is low effort and allows you to attend to other simple tasks at the same time. It is constantly finding patterns, making decisions, and simplifying the world.

System 2 takes a lot more effort but it can spot that the plate is by the oven and suggest it might not be a good idea to pick it up. It can attend to the vomit on the floor and gather clues from the nature of the vomit as to what might be the cause. It will halt conversation in the car when another car pulls out on you and it can interrupt the automatic reading of a story when you suddenly realise you forgot a critical step in your surgery earlier that day.

System 1 is fast and easy and takes little effort but it has its faults. It will answer a difficult question with an easier answer resulting in a gap. A good example to try is this simple question, try answering it quickly. A bat and ball cost £1.10. The bat costs £1 more than the ball. How much is the ball? If you reduce 'tools' to a hammer everything starts to look like a nail and although it works well most of the time it fails some of the time and is probably not optimum most of the time. The answer is not 10p.

7.2 Don't Let Procrustes Get Hold of Occam's Razor

William of Ockham was a fourteenth-century Bishop, Philosopher and Theologian. He proposed that when determining causation entities must not be multiplied beyond necessity, his so called Principle of Parsimony. In other words, if the patient has a headache, watery eyes and a sore throat it is likely that they have a common cold, rather than a brain tumour, lacrimal duct tumour and reflux from a gastric tumour. Alternatively, Hickam's dictum stated that 'A man can have as many diseases as he damn well pleases'. You will recall the common advice to medical students, 'If you hear the sound of hooves think horses not zebras'. This fits well with System 1 thinking unless you forgot you are in Kruger Park or that Zebras had recently escaped from a nearby Zoo. Exceptions do occur and Hickam will be correct some of the time. It's 5p by the way.

Procrustes was an Inn Keeper in ancient Greece before the days of 'trip advisor', regretfully. He would allow you to have a bed for the night but if your legs were too long (I am safe there), he would cut them down to fit the bed. Diagnostically and surgically we all run this risk of forcing the fit.

In medicine in general and in surgery specifically, the surgeon is looking for simple solutions and, from 'Part II', hopefully 'Lean' solutions. However, there is a danger that the solution is overly simple and even wrong but expediency and simplicity have trumped diligence and rigour and suddenly and conveniently the problem fits the solution. There is a danger that Procrustes will get hold of Occam's razor and screws start to look a bit like nails (all be it with some funny ridges) but we can forget about those and simply hammer harder. System 1 wants to get hold of the razor and give it to Procrustes however, in experienced hands, the decisions made in System 1 are usually correct.

I think that simply being aware of these two systems is of benefit in surgery although in reality, in the heat of the moment, when this type of System 1 reasoning leads to an error, it is unlikely to be correctly identified at the time (Croskerry et al. 2013). Having spent a year preparing this book, swimming and marinading in its ideas, I came foul of this twice over the last month. One time resulted in an additional expense the other time in a complication. During a case it is likely the surgeon with experience will be operating predominantly in System 1 and the trainee in System 2, both very appropriately. For training purposes, it is important to be rigorous and reflective in the learning phase as these manoeuvres and techniques will move into System 1 over time. For the experienced surgeon access to System 2 requires analysis post operatively, in space and time and requires effort. For the trainee, System 2 surgery is hard work and tiring and the concentration required will prevent them from building up an overall understanding of the surgery. This is OK. Over time the manoeuvres will move into System 1 and then attention can be given to the whys and where's and eventually threat detection and prevention of errors.

This is where I find teaching surgeons to be of specific benefit *to me*. The Afrikaans word to '*Learn*' is '*Leer*' and it is the same as the word to 'Teach'. Why Afrikaans suddenly? Bernard Wolff, a very good friend and former colleague from my fellowship in Melbourne, is South African and we still talk regularly about tricky cases. We both still want to learn (and teach) after 14 years. Debriefing after surgery with trainees facilitates System 2 thinking for both parties. If you have ever tried to explain why you did a complex case a certain way to a trainee you will understand the immense unpacking required and perhaps why our brains choose to favour System 1 thinking. If the ball is 5p, then the bat is £1.05 (£1 more) and the total is £1.10.

7.3 Cognitive Load Theory (CLT) and Expert Versus Novice Distinctions (Sweller 1988)

CLT was developed by Sweller in 1988 and is based on resource limited theory and schema theory. It is useful to briefly review this work as it helps us to understand the differences seen between novice and expert problem solvers and perhaps, trainees from experienced consultants. Sweller identified three key differences between experts and novices when solving complex problems.

7.4 Memory of Problem State Configurations

Looking at problem solving in chess masters and less experienced players, his work found that the only real difference between the two groups occurred in the memory of realistic chess positions. Both remembered realistic chess positions and sequences of moves in chunks but the chunks of the masters were far larger than those of the novices. This effect was abolished when using random positions suggesting this had little to do with short-term memory. Masters can take in the board and recognise realistic chess positions and the required numerous sequences of moves to succeed. In a similar way an experienced surgeon will often have an instant plan when faced with a complex case but a junior will think through each step.

7.5 Problem-Solving Strategies

Transformation problems consist of an initial state, a goal state and legal problem-solving operators. Most mathematics problems and, I would suggest, surgical problems can be classified as such. Work with physics problems suggested that novices tended to use means-ends analysis, working backward from the goal and setting subgoals until equations containing no unknowns other than the desired subgoal were found. Then the sequence could be reversed and a forward working sequence followed to solve the problem. In contrast, experts began by choosing an equation which allowed a value for an unknown to be calculated and then continued until the other unknowns were calculated and the goal was achieved. Experts work forwards recognising each problem from previous experience using schemas. A schema is a structure that allows problems to be categorised and then the sequence of moves required to solve this can be brought to mind. This is also seen in 'speed cubers'. They recognise the pattern and then fire almost automatic sequences of moves faster than they can see and assess, hence they can do this when blindfolded. In the same way an experienced surgeon will recognise a complex situation as another schema with an inbuilt set of goals and with the steps required to solve it. They can thus default to System 1 thinking which also reduces cognitive load and allows them to attend to other aspects of the surgery further benefitting the flow of surgery, like preventing complications before they arise.

7.6 Features Used in Categorising Problems

Sweller found that experts tended to group problems on the basis of the solution mode whereas novices tended to group problems according to the surface structures such as the inclusion of shared objects in the problem statement. Experts keep the big picture in mind, novices focus in on the detail. I recently debriefed one of my

Fellows who had attempted a difficult case alone. He was well aware the case was on the edge of his comfort and competence zone and had recorded the surgery and planned to debrief with me. What was interesting, as I watched his surgery, was that I could see why he had done what he had done, each step made sense. However, he had not correctly identified the overall aim of his surgery which was not actually success *this time* but rather to fail well, allowing inflammation to settle and then setting up the next surgery for success. His attention to the surface elements of the problem did not allow him to see the bigger picture and so his well-executed steps took him in the wrong direction.

Abernethy presented findings based on work looking at the characteristics of experts and how this might improve the effectiveness of training in any sphere. Abernethy described several characteristics of experts including having a rich mental library of images and patterns; being good at grouping together the components of complex movements ('chunking'); performing simple tasks at a subconscious level ('on automatic pilot'), allowing attention to be better focussed towards recognising and adjusting to varying or abnormal circumstances and getting better feedback so that small mistakes were recognised and corrected along the way (Abernethy 2001). This certainly resonates with my experience in surgery and is consistent with the work of Sweller and Kahneman.

There is some evidence from CLT that conventional problem-solving activity is not effective in schema acquisition, perhaps further explaining why my Fellow got into difficulty. The significant cognitive load required for solving problems step by step means there is not enough bandwidth to acquire schemas at the same time. The cognitive processes required for each are also different with little overlap and further, some forms of problem solving actually interfere with learning which may be an issue with the use of simulators in surgical training. Work by Sweller and Levine explored puzzles that could be solved either by a means of end analysis or by inducing a rule based on the problem structure. Puzzles were easily solved using means end analysis but the rules were not discovered in the process unless significant additional material was provided. This was further supported by giving maze problems to two groups; one group knew the goal state and could solve in a forward direction but the other group was not given the goal, they had to find both the goal and the route to the goal. The latter group was able to deduce the structural characteristics required to solve the maze whereas the first group could not, preventing them from even solving some simple mazes (Sweller and Levine 1982). Surgery is very similar. We tend to teach the trainee one step at a time and focus on each step. This is especially evident with the use of simulators early on but it is easy to get lost in the detail and not see the overall direction required to ultimately solve the problem. I certainly remember feeling like an automaton early on in my training simply following each step given by the boss but with no real idea of why or where we were heading in the surgery.

If we go back to my analogy of reading in 'Part I'. We all learn to read by learning the sounds of individual letters and groups of letters and then blending sounds to make words. At this stage no information is taken on board, they are sounded words with no meaning. As the reader progresses the sounds and blends become second nature and then the reader can start to pay attention to the meaning of the words in each sentence. With more time and experience sense can be made of paragraphs, chapters and eventually entire books extracting deeper meaning, motives and lessons. The genre of a book can be quickly ascertained. Surgery requires a heavy cognitive load in the first instance and progress is slow, this is System 2 at work. Holding instruments, moving them and tissue manipulation all have to be mastered in System 2 and then slowly put into System 1. Once in System 1 the manoeuvres no longer take up much bandwidth or cognitive load and instead attention can now be safely directed to bigger goals, sequences of moves of increasing complexity until ultimately an entire schema is formed, even for apparently complex situations, with plenty of bandwidth to watch for variation and avoiding complications.

7.7   Flow State

System 1 surgery, functioning appropriately, is perhaps analogous to 'Flow state'. Flow is the state of mind in which a person is fully engaged in an activity often oblivious to time (Csikszentmihalyi 1990). Flow state has been shown to be an effective state for surgeons to achieve (Ahlborg et al. 2012, 2015). Yu compared and contrasted CLT to flow state arguing that in flow state surgeons perform at their best improving the effectiveness of the operation and improving patient safety. However, if challenge begins to exceed skill this flow state is lost and anxiety increases but if the task begins fall well below the skill level of the surgeon, boredom ensues (Yu et al. 2022). Unfortunately, as is common in this literature, this study involved medical students, not experienced surgeons, perhaps limiting a more specific application.

My best days in theatre are almost certainly in flow state. Time passes quickly, cases go well, everyone seems happy and even after a long day tiredness is not an issue. This could be flow state or simply System 1 operating appropriately and with cognitive ease. Interestingly I see this state often in life, it is when children are at play!

To finish, and for some lighter relief, let me return to our favoured comparison, aviation. I interviewed The Captain on the subject of problem solving and it provided a fascinating insight into key differences between the two professions in this regard. Part of the conversation I have already covered in Chap. 6 on the effect of culture on failure but we also explored the extremes of problems solving in aviation from highly predictable problems with advanced decisions made during various briefs through to the sudden problem and finally the 'mayday' situation.

7.8   Solutions Before Manifestation—'Problem Solving in Advance'

Some problems can be identified in advance using checklists or briefs. In aviation there are three briefs. The first is carried out in the terminal building, the second on the flight deck pre-take-off and the third around thirty minutes before descent, the approach brief. The pre-flight briefs include aspects of the plane and its fitness to fly, the load expected, the weather at take-off, destination and on route and subsequently, the fuel required allowing for contingencies. The Captain reviews flight plan data and weather data which can be assimilated quickly with his experience although, consistent with the Dunning Kruger effect (later), sometimes he is more concerned rather than less as he computes the interactions of various factors. Aircraft carry 5 min of extra fuel as standard but he needs to decide if this is sufficient and this will depend on several factors especially the weather at the destination and the risk of a re-route last minute. I suggested that I would expect the least experienced pilots to take the most fuel and there was some agreement with this observation. Pilots are ranked and outliers are reviewed as an ongoing process. Fuel is expensive.

In surgery we also have several briefs as part of the WHO surgical safety checklist which occur pre-anaesthesia, pre-incision and before the patient leaves the operating theatre. The key issues to identify for surgical care include confirmation of identity of the patient and intended procedure, kit requirements and any potential patient issues with allergies, airway, etc. In theatre the intended procedure and any variations are discussed as well as the sterility of kit, imaging, etc. Finally, as the patient leaves the theatre the final checklist confirms the procedure actually performed and any instructions as well as ensuring the kit is complete.

I do not analyse the case via these checks, this happens on the pre-operative ward round if not well before depending on complexity or novelty. Although no plan survives first contact with the enemy it is wise to have plan with complex or novel cases utilising System 2 thinking. However, many cases receive little or no additional attention as they are 'routine' in my mind. I assume System 1 thinking. I might discuss outliers with the anaesthetist but the vast majority would proceed as routine with no exceptional communication. The aim of both briefs is to identify potential problems before we start and surgery has learned a lot from aviation in this regard although the actual checks do not seem terribly comparable in application with some criticism, they are in danger of becoming 'tick box' exercises.

7.9   Solutions During Manifestations—'Problem Solving in Real Time'

At the level before 'catastrophic' the pilots have various frameworks that guide thinking. These frameworks allow psychological control to be established and enable clear communication, remember there are always two pilots in the cockpit. Following the emergence of the problem, the pilots will 'FNC' it 'Fly, Navigate and Communicate'. The Captain stated that when something goes wrong, the temptation is to do something and this 'FNC' gives the pilots that something to do rather than make a hasty and likely poor decision. The plane needs to keep flying, whether by auto pilot or manual, and needs to be going in the correct direction (F and N) allowing time to communicate (C). Having 'FNC'd' it, attention is paid to the on-board computer system, the electronic centralised aircraft monitor or ECAM. This will give the pilots information and instructions on dealing with the issue, planes can help the pilot here significantly. Surgeons get no help from the equipment and are often alone. Then another framework is employed like 'TDODAR' (Time, Diagnosis, Options, Decide, Act/Assign, Review) with more communication and shared problem solving as they move the problem through the framework. It really struck me that it is not left to pilot experience and competence alone, these frameworks enable combined problem solving, sharing of workload, division of labour, maintenance of psychological state, equality of input and a review loop built in to assess for change. Surgery is not at all like this. In surgery a sudden event is not dealt with within any framework I am aware of. It is up to the surgeon to deal with it and usually alone. The general advice is to stop and think and plan. If time is not an issue, then I would tend to try to understand the underlying problem and then scenario plan in my mind various solutions and expected outcomes and consequences of the actions drawing heavily on my experience. Experience plays a critical role in dealing with these events as previous scenarios and outcomes are brought to mind as per the schema theory discussed above. It feels very much on the shoulders of the surgeon with their experience and knowledge the key to solving the problem. This may also feed into the blame versus no blame cultures with problem solving in aviation a collaborative exercise with shared responsibility but in surgery, a lone exercise with personal responsibility? Pilots are also prepared for such stressful situations during their regular simulator training. They are pushed up to and beyond their limit deliberately so that they can recognise what their limit feels like. It might be dry mouth; it might be sweating or a pit in the stomach and recognising what the signal is allows communication of the internal state between pilots avoiding further psychological overload. As we discussed in Part I, simulator training for surgeons is stress free, we will only experience this stress in the moment and cannot train well for it.

7.10   Solutions During Crisis—'Advanced Problem Solving in No Time'

At the other end of the spectrum is the 'Mayday' event. This is a very high stress, high consequence and thankfully rare event. There is no equivalent for surgeons given the potential for significant loss of life, including that of the pilots and crew. Perhaps the most famous incident was Captain Sully's landing on the Hudson. Sully, held up as a hero by the press, humbly denied this status putting it down to those who had gone before, teamwork and training, although he had apparently visualised just such a scenario (Think back to imagery from Part I). He remained calm, made decisions in communication with his co-pilot following the well-trodden frameworks and landed the plane. Commenting in an interview after the event he had this to say about his actions. "One way of looking at this might be that for 42 years, I've been making small, regular deposits in this bank of experience, education and training. And on January 15, the balance was sufficient so that I could make a very large withdrawal" His humility is evident however his experience cannot be ignored.

7.11   Conclusion

System 1 is where experienced surgeons function most of the time and this is entirely appropriate, most of the time. With experience comes the formation of schemas allowing problems to be quickly recognised and entire sequences of surgical manoeuvres selected and executed. Cognitive load is reduced and attention can be paid to other aspects of surgery which allows for higher volumes of surgeries to be completed safely with the extra bandwidth available to look for and prevent complications. It can allow the surgeon to interact with staff and the patient, improving the overall experience of the surgery for both these parties. Although entirely appropriate to be in System 1, the experienced surgeon would be well advised to access System 2 intermittently in order to seek to improve further given that System 1 works well most of the time but not all the time. Finally, given the high cognitive load of the trainee operating in System 2 a thorough debrief is best undertaken after surgery, with or without coffee, and who knows it might result in your writing a book.

7.12   To Try

Record three cases and or review three cases in depth, preferably one with a complication.

When was System 1 in operation?

When was System 2 in operation if at all? Solving the complication?

Challenge your thinking and replay with a different approach using System 2, is it better?

Find an experienced surgeon, give them the case details and ask how they would proceed tapping into *their* System 1 and System 2 thinking.

Can you learn from their approach, might they learn from your approach?

How might an understanding of CLT change the way you train or learn?

References

Abernethy AB. Learning from experts: how the study of expertise might help design more effective training. In: Proceedings of the 37th annual conference of the ergonomics Society of Australia; 2001.

Ahlborg L, Hedman L, Rasmussen C, Felländer-Tsai L, Enochsson L. Non-technical factors influence laparoscopic simulator performance among OBGYN residents. Gynecol Surg. 2012;9(4):415–20. https://doi.org/10.1007/s10397-012-0748-2.

Ahlborg L, Weurlander M, Hedman L, Nisell H, Lindqvist PG, Felländer-Tsai L, Enochsson L. Individualized feedback during simulated laparoscopic training: a mixed methods study. Int J Med Educ. 2015;6:93–100. https://doi.org/10.5116/ijme.55a2.218b.

Croskerry P, Singhal G, Mamede S. Cognitive debiasing 1: origins of bias and theory of debiasing. BMJ Qual Safety, 2013;22(Suppl 2), ii58–64. https://doi.org/10.1136/bmjqs-2012-001712.

Csikszentmihalyi M. Flow: the psychology of optimal experience. Harper and Row; 1990.

Kahneman D. Thinking fast and slow. In: Farrar, SG. Editors. Penguin; 2011.

Sweller J. Cognitive load during problem solving: effects on learning. Cogn Sci. 1988;12(2):257–85. https://doi.org/10.1207/s15516709cog1202_4.

Sweller J, Levine M. Effects of goal specificity on means–ends analysis and learning. J Exp Psychol Learn Mem Cogn. 1982;8(5):463–74. https://doi.org/10.1037/0278-7393.8.5.463.

Yu P, Pan J, Wang Z, Shen Y, Li J, Hao A, Wang H. Quantitative influence and performance analysis of virtual reality laparoscopic surgical training system. BMC Med Educ. 2022;22(1):92. https://doi.org/10.1186/s12909-022-03150-y.

Chapter 8
Heuristics and Cognitive Bias—What Can We Learn from Waking Up?

In surgery, don't take short cuts and don't take long cuts, stay on the well-trodden path there are snakes in the grass

—Stephen Lash

It's ok to drive home and not remember how you got there. However, It's inconvenient to arrive at the shops having planned to go home.

—Stephen Lash

Abstract The world is complex. We have developed ways of understanding, interpreting and responding to this complex environment using shortcuts. These shortcuts reduce our cognitive load and thus enable us to detect potential threats and respond. These shortcuts are called heuristics and they are very powerful. Heuristics do reduce task complexity, facilitating rapid judgement and responses, but they also result in gaps between the normative behaviour predicted and the heuristically determined behaviour observed. Cognitive biases can result from these shortcuts and interfere with good decision making. Heuristics are predominantly, but not exclusively, a System 1 tool. Although these heuristics do work well in the hands of experts, they can also be the source of prejudice, cognitive bias and, at times, bad decisions. I will review the main heuristics and cognitive biases I see relevant to surgery and suggest modifications to clinical audit as a result. I will also explore the literature on cognitive debiasing and apply it to the practice of surgery. Can we avoid the likely errors when making decisions using heuristics?

Keywords Surgical heuristics · Cognitive bias · System 1 thinking · System 2 thinking · Representative heuristic · Anchoring heuristic · Availability heuristic · Risk aversion · Loss aversion · Prospect theory

8.1   Introduction

The world is complex. We have developed ways of understanding, interpreting and responding to this complex environment using shortcuts. These shortcuts reduce our cognitive load and thus enable us to detect potential threats and respond. These shortcuts are called heuristics and they are very powerful. Heuristics do reduce task complexity, facilitating rapid judgement and responses, but they also result in gaps between the normative behaviour predicted and the heuristically determined behaviour observed (Kahneman et al. 1982). Cognitive biases can result from these shortcuts and interfere with good decision making. In the 1940s Simon coined the term 'Satisficing' to denote a process whereby a decision is judged as 'good enough', although it could be optimised with more time and effort (Simon 1947). In essence satisficing is a type of heuristic. We have all 'satisficed' when looking for a new house, a new kitchen appliance or making a diagnosis. As new options come up, we make judgements on what each aspect has in favour of proceeding and what aspects count against and then weigh each factor until such point that the perceived level of satisfaction exceeds current requirements. It is sufficient and it satisfies even though it could be optimised with a lot more time and effort. In the early 1970s Tversky and Kahneman further explored and defined heuristics in human decision making winning a Nobel prize for their work. I will draw mainly from their work as we apply heuristics to surgery. Heuristics enable us to apply previous knowledge to new situations and require little mental energy. They are predominantly, but not exclusively, a System 1 tool. Although these heuristics do work well in the hands of experts, they can also be the source of prejudice, cognitive bias and, at times, bad decisions. As surgeons, we want, and perhaps need, to function on 'automatic pilot' most of the time such that we have sufficient bandwidth to remain vigilant for potential complications. By becoming aware of these heuristics and cognitive biases we might be able to learn from them, challenge them and hopefully become better surgeons. I will review the main heuristics and cognitive biases I see relevant to surgery and suggest modifications to clinical audit as a result. I will also explore the literature on cognitive debiasing and apply it to the practice of surgery. Can we avoid these errors when making decisions using heuristics? Three heuristics were initially described by Kahneman and Tversky; representative, anchoring and availability heuristics.

8.2   Representative Heuristic

The representative heuristic results in the tendency to classify objects, people, events, etc., into categories. The simplification of the world into relatively few categories helps us to make quick decisions but it is low resolution and lacks nuance. It is associated with prototype theory whereby we tend to group objects into categories forming a prototype. The more the object of current regard matches the prototype the more confident we are it belongs to that category. I see this regularly at work in the diagnosis of disease and its subsequent management. I discussed schema theory previously, likely functioning on this heuristic. However, the specific set of issues might not be fully represented by the prototype and errors can result. Remember, System 1 thinking wants to answer difficult questions with easier answers.

8.3   Anchoring Heuristic

When people make choices, they tend to depend more heavily on pre-existing information or the first information they come across. This is known as anchoring bias. If I were to suggest the complication rate of technique 'A' was around 50% to a group of medical students, and then asked them what the actual percentage was they are likely to start at 50% and then adjust it to arrive at their answer. However, if I suggested the complication rate of technique 'A' was 0.5% to a different group of medical students, they will likely start at 0.5% and increase the rate somewhat. It is extremely unlikely the two figures will be similar as each group will anchor on the first number given. This is a powerful heuristic and, in my experience, is often very difficult to expose even if you know about it. Assumptions go deep and are rarely challenged and are even subsequently reinforced.

8.4   Availability Heuristic

The bias of availability occurs when we take into account an extreme or notable event, a recent experience, or something that's particularly vivid to us, to make our judgements. This heuristic is very common in surgery and tends to anchor on failure because a complication is memorable whereas routine surgery is forgotten. The 'one that went wrong' is powerful in influencing future surgery because we fear failure (Part II). I will discuss later how losses 'hurt more' than successes 'feel good' in exploring loss aversion, risk aversion and prospect theory and demonstrate how each contribute to and augment, this heuristic. Prospective and retrospective audit go some way to providing actual data to mitigate this heuristic although beware of the 'law of small numbers', which I will also discuss later. Being aware of the availability heuristic enables the surgeon to challenge its conclusions and avoids a surgical technique that changes every case.

8.5   Examples in Surgery

8.5.1   Representative Heuristic

I have certainly come into difficulty with this at times. I can easily recall a specific case (availability heuristic!) that went badly. The case was identical to and therefore 'representative' of many others I had done before however, I failed to take into account one small aspect that made the case unlike all the others. A significant head tremor, that had not been obvious in clinic, became very obvious as the patient laid down under the operating microscope! System 1 was in full operation; auto pilot was on and the schema was loaded and ready to go. I had answered a more difficult question with an easier answer. The case was difficult and the result suboptimal. On her second eye I used an alternative and much easier technique successfully. Not having multiple approaches and techniques can further drive this heuristic, hammers, nails, razors and Procrustes once more. However, as a counterbalance to multiple techniques, one must also take into account learning curves and general competence (Part I). "Sure, we want a quiver full of arrows but they all have to fire straight and further, regrettably, not all of us are William Tell". Schemas have to be built up slowly over many years and refined and challenged intermittently, as new technology or knowledge becomes available, using System 2 thinking. Deciding on a schema too early, or trusting a schema too long, falling fowl of the representative heuristic, is likely to result in suboptimal performance and worse outcomes.

8.5.2   Anchoring

I see anchoring at work from the administration of lists to the actual practice of surgery. One example of anchoring at the administrative level would be the number of surgeries carried out on an NHS list. Be it gastroscopies, knee replacements or, for this discussion, cataract surgery we anchor on a number. For many years that number has been around 6–8 cases in a four-hour session with two sessions per day. Even this basic organisation of lists is also likely the result of anchoring. Why four hours? Why time? Why not productivity? As a consequence, a surgeon completing 10 cases would be seen as efficient and competent and 5 could be easily explained away. The systems and processes embed around this number; expectations are set and the anchors descend. Bureaucracy develops around the system; the safety culture sets expectations and norms and everything is subsequently taught to the next generation and the anchors sink even deeper. However, more recently, independent sector surgeons in the UK are completing 15 cases on a list. I have heard two challenges to this in NHS departments I have worked in, either that the cases are easier, the so called 'cherry picking' argument or the inference that these surgeons or businesses must be cutting corners, a 'safety' argument. Most of these independent sector surgeons are NHS surgeons by the way. However, if we move to another country, with different attitudes to safety, bureaucracy, administration and the division of labour the numbers can be *many orders* of magnitude greater. Dr Akahoshi Takayuki in Japan performs around 60 cases per day for example. Although he may only be very slightly faster than very good UK surgeons, it is clear he does *nothing* except operate on his lists with many of the administrative and preparatory tasks done by others. The Aravind Hospital in India is another example. It has a fraction of the safety measures we have in the West but outperforms us in terms of number of patients operated on in a day and with lower infection rates (Chang 2019). Exposing systems to other cultures, countries or disciplines can be very powerful in exposing anchoring.

The snowball technique (Part II) is a version of anchoring on a surgical 'micro-technical scale'. Here an adverse event is compensated for by *adding* in safety measures. The subtle anchor on safety is that 'more' must be safer. I used the example of the main section and side port in cataract surgery as my example. However, it is much harder to *stop* doing something once you have added it in. This is driven by other heuristics like the availability heuristic, risk aversion, loss aversion as well as prospect theory which I will explore shortly. This is where sitting with another surgeon, preferably in another system or even country may help to reveal the anchors and challenge them. As opposed to 'adding' the other form of anchoring involves 'sticking'. Surgeons can anchor on their techniques which can result in stagnation rather than expansion both in terms of the individual surgeon and surgery itself. Again, this behaviour can be driven by the availability heuristic, risk aversion, loss aversion and prospect theory.

8.6 Risk Aversion, Prospect Theory and Loss Aversion

Given the conclusions from my chapter on failure (Part II), it is easy to see why risk aversion is so prevalent in society and specifically in surgery today. The cost of failure can be high (Richardson 2022). However, risk aversion comes with a cost. It leads to paying a premium to avoid uncertainty, think of all your insurance policies. Risk aversion is also very important when consenting patients for surgery. They need to understand what will happen if nothing is done and understand that doing nothing (perhaps the default position of an anxious patient who fears surgery), comes with risks. Risk is everywhere and unavoidable and we need to balance the risk. Fearful patients often pay a higher cost, by refusing earlier surgery, in the end.

Kahneman and Tversky developed Prospect theory in 1979 and found that losses hurt more than the equivalent gains (Kahneman and Tversky 1979). Their theory challenged expected utility theory which would suggest that decision makers behave in a totally rational manner, and described how people actually behave. We feel 'sadder' about *losing* ten pounds than 'happier' at *finding* ten pounds. Prospect theory suggests a loss of $1000 can only be truly offset by a gain of $2000 in some individuals. It helps to explain why gamblers often get into more trouble as they repeatedly try to gamble their way out of losses. Applied to surgery, a failure is going to feel 'bad' more than a success is going to feel 'good', hence surgeons may tend towards avoiding failure even if this comes at a cost. In my personal reflection on my first year as a consultant, I tended towards overtreatment, the cost paid by the patient in terms of hospital visits and perhaps comfort and by the system in terms of a higher cost of treatment.

Loss aversion is often stronger than the motivation to obtain a goal. I see this when trying to teach a new technique to a trainee who has become comfortable in their present technique or when I become aware of a new technique that may be better than a technique I am used to. It's hard to stray outside the comfort zone. Being 'in training' is the perfect time to learn new approaches, to imitate the current boss with the expectation that failure will occur but under the consultant's safety net. However, for the experienced surgeon settling too soon might cause problems later on as technology advances. How often might more experienced surgeons satisfice rather than maximise, how often might they avoid the difficult procedure in favour of the more comfortable procedure for fear of complications? Learning new techniques involves a learning curve, increased complications and increased risk in the short term as well as difficulty and effort. Our default is not to venture into new territory and yet we need to push into this fear for surgery to develop both personally and as a discipline. I do wonder how we would get open heart surgery off the ground in the West today. We stand on the shoulders of the risk takers who went before us. Somehow, experienced surgeons need to maintain a 'persistent learning state' which may also facilitate the introduction of surgical coaches discussed in 'Part I'.

8.7   The Law of Small Numbers

The law of small numbers suggests that extreme results can be more or less common when the sample size is small. When combined with risk aversion and the availability heuristic, surgeons will tend to remember the exceptional case that went badly out of the relatively small case series and take steps to prevent it happening again. Individual surgeons cannot generate the volumes required for thorough assessment and evidence-based practice to avoid the law of small numbers; we really need big data. I am sure we have all had clinics where every other patient appears to be a complication. It is easy to lose heart with small numbers or conversely feel invincible with apparent 100% success rates.

8.7.1   Availability Heuristic

Having explored risk aversion, loss aversion, prospect theory and the law of small numbers I can better explore surgical examples of the availability heuristic which is perhaps the most powerful in operation surgically. As I discussed, the bias of availability occurs when we take into account an extreme or notable event, a recent experience, or something that's particularly vivid to us, to make our judgements. Given that prospect theory has found that losses (failures) hurt more than gains (successes) feel good it is reasonable to conclude that failures are usually more notable and vivid to the surgeon than successes and therefore more likely to be remembered, forming the substrate of the availability heuristic. In other words, this heuristic is likely to be overly represented in the realm of failure. If we add to this the heuristics of loss aversion and risk aversion especially in combination with the law of small numbers one can understand how these might drive behaviour in surgeons who are trying hard not to fail. Confirmation bias can also come into play reinforcing the decisions made. This was certainly my experience in the first year of my consultant post. The more I intervened the more it made sense to continue to intervene as all the retinas were flat!

As a Fellow my complications (few in number) stayed behind as I moved onto the next rotation in a new hospital. As a new consultant the complications (*still* few in number if you please!) stayed with me and there were times it felt like every patient in a clinic was a complication. I remember chatting with the Fellows explaining that becoming a consultant is like becoming a trawler fishing captain where the only fish left in the net are the memorable, big (complicated) ones as all the small nimble (uncomplicated) fishes swim away! It is easy to see how small numbers can lead to an overestimation of complications and a feeling of ineptitude or conversely, zero complications and apparent surgical superpowers. The truth lies between the two and it's important not to change practice based on small numbers and the availability heuristic. This has interesting consequences for clinical audit.

8.8 Application—Clinical Audit—Prospective, Retrospective, Micro to Macro

The central quest of this book is what makes a good surgeon and what makes them better. When it comes to audit, the previous section on heuristics and System thinking suggest some practical changes as to how we audit in order to extract maximum benefit and become better surgeons. I will also draw upon some to the conclusions from 'Part II' with the chapters on 'failure' and 'lean' and invite similar reflection and analysis on multiple levels.

At the 'micro-technique' level, a 'mental reflection' audit at the end of each subsection of surgery is powerful in terms of achieving marginal gains. Marginal gains enable slow progress towards perfect execution. Micro-level analysis is low risk in terms of significant failure or complications and it facilitates 'Kaizen' and the practice of 'Lean' surgery (Part I). Along with 'goal setting theory', it can provide the substrate for detailed 'imagery', a technique that allows the surgeon to practise in their mind with actual improvement in subsequent motor performance through neuroplasticity. This level is critical in initial training or learning a new technique but it is also of value to the experienced surgeon looking to refine their skills.

At the procedural level, reflection and audit following each case allows access to System 2 thinking where challenge can be brought to bear on the System 1 solution already delivered. This is often better when discussed in a team or with another colleague (over coffee!) but can be a lone practice. Was there a better way?

At the next level, prospective audit allows the outcomes to be tracked on a case-by-case basis with memory of the actual surgery still relatively fresh. The surgeon can once more review their System 1 surgery and apply System 2 in the calm light of day with the outcome now manifest and question, assess and perhaps improve. Although I would highly recommend prospective audit, the surgeon needs to be aware of the availability heuristic, the law of small numbers and confirmation bias and NOT change practice every week unless a pattern of complications is manifest (although beware of the clustering effect!).

At the final level of reflection, once a year, NHS surgeons are required to report annual, retrospective, audits. These audits are very useful in terms of reducing the law of small numbers to a degree although 'big data' and national audits are far more powerful in this respect. It is at this stage that the surgeon can review aspects of practice and make small changes at the schema level. Analysis at this level is too remote and distant to improve micro-technique and so the levels and cycles repeat.

8.9 Surgical Heuristics?

Having reviewed the academic foundations of heuristics there is work applying heuristics specifically to surgery. Patkin discussed three types of heuristic in surgery; motor, perceptual and cognitive (Patkin 2008). Motor heuristics included how to actually grasp tissues and tricks of the trade for dissection. He acknowledged that these are very difficult for the trainee to pick up on even when made explicit and required identification, imitation and repetition to embed (Patkin 2008). This tends to support my thoughts on imagery and rehearsal from 'Part I'. No matter how hard you 'observe' you really need to actually 'do' in order to refine movements. I have experienced this when learning a new technique or teaching a new technique to a trainee. On trying to learn a specific novel technique, no matter how much I used imagery and reviewed the video footage in immense detail trying to make the micro-technique explicit, I could only make progress by actually doing it. Patkin also suggested that motor heuristics acted as an early warning system when tissues did not respond the way they usually did and enabled appropriate handling going forward. Patkin described perceptual heuristics as learning to see the surgical field as a surgeon. A simple walk through a city will be reported on very differently by a developer, an architect and an artist. Each will see what they look for and look for what they know. Patkin suggested that learning to view the surgical field as a surgeon required a lot of time. This makes sense given that a more junior trainee will be operating in System 2 with a high cognitive load much of the time and oblivious to the nuances of the surgical field as they focus on the actual task in hand. In many specialities a viewing system is used to view the surgical field, be this a microscope, loupes or a laparoscopic system. The use of these systems needs to become automatic in order to allow attention to the surgical field. Finally, Patkin described cognitive heuristics as the planning of movements ensuring, for example, that the surgeon measured twice and cut once as well as planning complex sequences of movement.

There are many other heuristics and cognitive biases and in the next section I will review those I feel are most useful to the surgeon.

8.10 The Sunk-Cost Fallacy

This fallacy occurs when people continue to invest additional resources into a losing account despite better investments being available. As a result, winning stocks are sold too early and losing stocks are held on too long. Escalating commitment drives this fallacy. There is something very difficult about stopping a course of treatment for a patient or even an operation midway through but sometimes this is exactly what should be done. Prospect theory explains why people in dire straits will tend to take gambles with a high chance of making things worse because of a small chance of avoiding a huge loss. When surgery is going badly it is important to consider stopping, if safe to do so, rather than making things much worse. As we explored in the 'Lean' chapter (Part II), errors often compound with interest. I have seen cases where the best option was to stop and end the surgery safely, rather than pursue a certain outcome at significant cost. I find stopping a fascinating topic. I have asked other consultants when they stop and generally get a 'never' followed by a thoughtful 'except when…!' I have had cases that have gone 'off piste' and I have persevered with a good outcome and others where I just sensed it was better to stop and come back another day. I cannot tell you why beyond some sixth sense or intuition, a feeling that there was a 'strong headwind' that day and 'nothing was working' or was this simply heuristics and bias in operation once more. In terms of physical performance, we all have 'bad days' be it music, sport or surgery.

8.11 Hindsight

Hindsight judges' decisions on eventual outcomes rather than the decision process being sound or not. Kahneman suggests that hindsight works out particularly badly for physicians who get blamed for good decisions that had poor outcomes (Kahneman 2011). Hindsight fosters risk aversion but also brings significant glory to individuals who have taken extreme risks but succeeded. System 2 review is different to hindsight and needs to occur with some immediacy and objectivity with attention to process. Hindsight is often well separated from the event and simply focusses on outcome. Another surgeon I highly respect once told me that the decision you made on the table was the correct one. Hindsight forgets all the nuances of the particular situation and information available, simply looking at the (usually poor) outcome. Of course, we can and should learn from previous surgery, but this must be through System 2 based on decisions and data not just hindsight based on outcome.

8.12   Regression to the Mean

Regression to the mean is both encouraging and discouraging to surgeons. Combined with the law of small numbers and the availability heuristic it is easy for a surgeon to believe they are at the top of their profession and become overconfident or believe they should give up due to incompetence. Cases that go well do not always do well and cases that have gone badly do not always do badly. It is frustrating and sobering that after 15 years as a consultant my results remain about where they always have been. The lack of progress is very frustrating and sobering as well as encouraging after a bad run!

8.13   Fundamental Attribution Error

This is important in failure and attitudes to failure, especially in others, and also feeds into the culture within medicine that is generally unforgiving of failure. I discussed typical 'corridor conversations' briefly in 'Part II'. "I think Dr X had 'Y' complication because they are inexperienced, or lazy, or have poor dexterity, or are careless", etc. However, when I take time to think about 'Y' complication I remember that I have had exactly the same complication. At this stage the temptation is to determine that there were good (external) reasons for the complication and so it was not really my fault anyway. We have all had someone cut in front of us in traffic and felt annoyed. We have all cut in front of others when were desperately trying to get somewhere. Beware of the fundamental attribution error and its corrosive effect on teams as well as pushing the surgeon into an external locus of control with the resultant inability to change or improve (Part II).

8.14   Dunning-Kruger Effect

The less you know the more confident you are. The more you know the less confident you are. This effect can be a barrier to training where I want to teach an alternative technique to a trainee or when I spot a complication approaching around the corner that they are blissfully unaware of but moving swiftly towards. It can be hard to take advice, even from an expert. As for the expert it perhaps explains the 'imposter syndrome' many of us feel at times. This is perhaps normal and actually reassuring preventing the slide into hubris.

8.15 Clustering Illusion

We find patterns and clusters in random data. This is very powerful surgically along with the law of small numbers. A random cluster can feel like the end of the world. All trainees, myself included, have suffered this and all I can do is reassure them (and myself at times) and encourage them to press on. Of course, there are times when this clustering is not an illusion but is real and audit is a useful tool in differentiating the two.

8.16 Zero Risk Bias

This states that we prefer to reduce small risks to zero even if we can reduce more risk overall with another option. This perhaps goes some way to explain what I see on an institutional level in the NHS where we would rather reduce the risk of patients under our care by fractions of a percentage towards zero, which takes up more and more time and energy, with processes generally added to, but ignore the subsequent expanding waiting list where patients are getting much worse, be it out of our sight, and will suffer more harm in the end. I discussed this 'see-saw' issue in 'Part II'. It also goes some way to explain the snowball technique whereby performing additional manoeuvres to reduce risk seems preferable to simply getting the first one right, reducing the overall risk of surgery.

Having explored the various heuristics and cognitive biases and their effects on our decisions, can we actually learn from them or even avoid them?

8.17 Recognizing Heuristics and Cognitive Bias in Clinical Decision Making. Can Intervention Reduce Errors?

Surgical care often requires fast decision making to save life and limb and the heuristics we have discussed are of great importance in facilitating this safe care and work well most of the time. However, these heuristics can also result in cognitive bias, incorrect conclusions and error (Hughes et al. 2020). In their paper, Antonacci et al. reviewed the impact of cognitive bias on the management of postoperative complications (Antonacci et al. 2021). They reported the incidence and distribution of various types of cognitive bias and evaluated their impact on the standard of care looking at 736 general surgical cases. They found that cognitive bias was attributed to around 33% of all cases with complications and found the most common (the terms 'heuristics' and 'cognitive bias' are used interchangeably) were anchoring, confirmation, omission, commission, overconfidence, premature closure, hindsight, diagnosis momentum, outcome and ascertainment bias. In another paper, looking at medical errors, the authors found that system related factors contributed to the diagnostic error in 65% of the cases and cognitive factors in 74% (Graber et al. 2005).

Heuristics and the subsequent biases are more common in System 1. Stanovich further elaborated on these System 1 processes according to their origins and described four main types (Stanovich 2010). Hard-wired or innate heuristics that may induce biases such as anchoring and adjustment, representativeness and availability heuristics. Processes regulated by our emotions, also hard-wired, such as happiness, sadness, fear, surprise, anger and disgust. Processes that become firmly embedded into our behavioural repertoire through overlearning in cultural and social domains and also in specific knowledge domains. And finally, processes that have developed through implicit learning. Formal training and education facilitate explicit knowledge however implicit knowledge develops through complex interactions, perceptions, attitude and complex relationships over time (Stanovich 2010). The hard-wired heuristics may be more difficult to overcome.

Croskerry presented two papers looking at the origins of cognitive bias and some potential interventions to reduce them (Croskerry et al. 2013a, b). Their work focussed on physicians rather than surgeons and also drew from the non-medical literature. As well as discussing the impact of various heuristics and cognitive biases they also discussed how other factors might make bias more likely including both external; team dynamics, environment, resources and internal; fatigue, sleep deprivation, cognitive load and personality. Some of these are very amenable to intervention. In his book, 'Why we Sleep', Matthew Walker described how surgeons who have had less than 6 h of sleep in the previous 24 were 170% more likely to have a serious complication (Walker 2017).

System 2 processes are also prone to biases although less commonly than System 1 processes. For example, when the stakes are high the usual processes are adapted, often resulting in the overestimate of a diagnosis, resulting in wasted resources rather than their optimal use and overtreatment. We are prone to both short cuts and long cuts and I certainly see this play out in surgery when the stakes are high and it is equally unhelpful, driven in part by loss aversion and fear of failure. Perhaps this is why it is not a good idea to treat a relative or a close friend?

Debiasing is part of everyday life and some are better than others at learning from previous actions and their consequences. Debiasing requires visibility and attention to the consequences of the action and a desire to rectify them. Going back to the concept of locus of control (LOC), an external LOC mindset is less likely to achieve debiasing given that the consequences of actions are often seen as outside the control of the person, simply chance and environment. I admitted that I had recently fallen foul of a System 1 error, effectively a representative heuristic, in spite of researching this book. The solution I instigated was a simple rhyme to chant under my breath which my scrub nurse has also picked up on with some amusement. It is unlikely I will make the same error again thanks to this simple intervention but it required an awareness of heuristics and bias, identifying the specific error and then applying an intervention. Various papers have explored the potential of debiasing using algorithms, the characteristics of decision makers and education.

Wilson and Brekke have suggested an algorithmic approach to debiasing. The algorithm described the actions once the bias is triggered starting with an awareness of the bias, the motivation to correct the bias, an awareness of the magnitude and direction of the bias, application of the appropriate debiasing strategy resulting in successful debiasing with the subsequent integration of the new learnings for future optimal decision making (Wilson and Brekke 1994). Bazerman suggested that the key to debiasing was some disequilibrium of the decision maker such that change was desired suggesting this may come about by being informed of a potential bias or discovering the adverse consequences of bias, particularly helped if there was an emotional component or the consequences were particularly vivid (Bazerman and Moore 2013). In this regard surgery is perhaps more potent than medicine with a more direct action-consequence paradigm; you cut the vessel it immediately bleeds and stress ensues. We have already discussed how many of the heuristics tend to operate in failure and so the incentive to 'debias' is perhaps more powerful in surgery once the surgeon is actually aware of this predominantly unconscious decision-making system.

Stanovich and West focussed on the characteristics of the decision maker in order to eliminate bias. The need for an awareness of the rules, procedures and strategies needed to overcome the bias, the ability to detect the bias and override it and finally to be cognitively capable of decoupling from the bias (Stanovich and West 2008). Stanovich also suggested that a critical feature of debiasing was the ability to suppress the automatic response from System 1 by decoupling it. 'The decision maker must be able to detect situational cues to detect the need to override the heuristic response and then analyse alternative solutions' (Stanovich 2011). However, I have some issues with 'in the moment debiasing' when applied to surgery as I will discuss later in this section.

In the second paper in their series, Croskerry described strategies for cognitive debiasing including education, to prevent errors in the future, workplace strategies to avoid bias in the moment and forcing strategies to make errors either impossible or very difficult to make. A barrier to the educational strategies was the observation that many doctors are in the 'pre-contemplative' phase with regard to heuristics and bias. I tend to agree hence writing this section. I am keen to make the reader aware of this area of decision making in surgery. The educational strategies aimed to reduce errors in the future and involved training in theories and reasoning in medical decision making through to computer based cognitive tutoring and simulation training (Croskerry et al. 2013b). They also reviewed specific strategies to prevent bias occurring in the moment and they admitted the evidence for these interventions is less than complete especially in medicine. Strategies relied on the application of System 2 (Type 2) thinking to the System 1 (Type 1) processes in operation. This was achieved by strategies such as slowing down, gathering more information, being more sceptical and even group decision strategies (Croskerry et al. 2013b). Although I believe their suggestions surrounding education are of great benefit to the surgeon, the 'in the moment' strategies are unlikely to work well in surgery and further, may result in more complications not less as the surgeon is forced out of System 1 thinking and, perhaps, 'Flow state' into a world of endless options and cognitive overload.

Not all agree that debiasing actually works. Berner suggested that once aware of biases, overconfidence in judgements and decisions may prevent debiasing (Berner and Graber 2008). It has also been argued that even being aware of biases does not guarantee debiasing will occur and there is much scepticism around making change in this area (Kahneman 2011; Wilson and Brekke 1994).

8.18   Summary—Practical Debiasing for Surgeons

To extrapolate the key messages from the debiasing literature and then apply them usefully and specifically to surgery, I would suggest the following attitudes and interventions. Firstly, to be aware of the existence of heuristics and the potential cognitive biases that result. Taking time to simply learn about them is important and I hope I have helped in this regard although it is only a start. We make good decisions as surgeons most of the time but not all of the time and so in order to refine, if we truly want to be great surgeons, we need to stop and reflect. We need to be enthusiastic about exposing the underlying heuristics and cognitive biases when they become manifest, often after a complication, and then challenge them using System 2 thinking after the event. These learnings need to be incorporated into practice going forward and might be as simple as a chant in our heads. I would not encourage real time attempts at debiasing during routine surgery. I suspect the cognitive load would be excessive and complications actually more likely as a result. However, it is totally appropriate and hopefully common practice for the surgeon to slow down, challenge thinking and even discuss with the team *during* a complication. This process will be necessarily slow and never complete but it will affect a direction of travel towards excellence. It will take enthusiasm and effort, a desire to get better and a high level of conscientiousness (Part III). It is going to take teamwork and colleagues who are willing to enter into the process with honesty and integrity and share bad experiences without judgement. It will require an internal locus of control to affect change and much patience. There is no magic here, there is no 'surgical hack'. It is time and effort but I think it is worth it. It is endlessly fascinating and challenging and makes surgery far more interesting than simply going through the motions in System 1 ad infinitum. We are surgeons not technicians.

8.19   To Try

Review several cases especially one with a complication.

Do you have examples of Anchoring, availability and representative heuristics? Were they more common in System 1 as predicted?

Which of the cognitive biases resonate and why? What were the cognitive biases in play during your cases?

What will you do about these heuristics and biases, can you 'debias'?

References

Antonacci AC, Dechario SP, Antonacci C, Husk G, Patel V, Nicastro J, Coppa G, Jarrett M. Cognitive bias impact on management of postoperative complications, medical error, and standard of care. J Surg Res. 2021;258:47–53. https://doi.org/10.1016/j.jss.2020.08.040.

Bazerman MH, Moore DA Judgement in managerial decision making (8th ed.). Wiley; 2013.

Berner ES, Graber ML. Overconfidence as a cause of diagnostic error in medicine. Am J Med. 2008;121(5):S2–23. https://doi.org/10.1016/j.amjmed.2008.01.001.

Chang D. Lesson from the world's greatest team of cataract surgeons. Cataract surgery: telling it like it is; 2019

Croskerry P, Singhal G, Mamede S. Cognitive debiasing 1: origins of bias and theory of debiasing. BMJ Qual Safety. 2013a;22(Suppl 2), ii58–64. https://doi.org/10.1136/bmjqs-2012-001712.

Croskerry P, Singhal G, Mamede S. Cognitive debiasing 2: impediments to and strategies for change. BMJ Qual Safety. 2013b;22(Suppl 2), ii65–72. https://doi.org/10.1136/bmjqs-2012-001713

Graber ML, Franklin N, Gordon R. Diagnostic error in internal medicine; n.d. https://jamanetwork.com/.

Hughes TM, Dossett LA, Hawley ST, Telem DA. Recognizing heuristics and bias in clinical decision-making. Ann Surg. 2020;271(5):813–4. https://doi.org/10.1097/SLA.0000000000003699.

Kahneman D, Slovic P, Tversky A, 1982. Judgment under uncertainty. In Kahneman D, Slovic P, Tversky A, Editors. Cambridge University Press. https://doi.org/10.1017/CBO9780511809477.

Kahneman D, Tversky A. Prospect theory: an analysis of decision under risk. Econometrica. 1979;47(2):263. https://doi.org/10.2307/1914185.

Kahneman, D. Thinking fast and slow. In Farrar SG, editors. Penguin; 2011.

Patkin M. Surgical heuristics. ANZ J Surg. 2008;78(12):1065–9. https://doi.org/10.1111/j.1445-2197.2008.04752.x.

Richardson J. 3 in 10 doctors fear being blamed or facing legal action after admitting mistakes. GP Online; 2022.

Simon HA. Administrative Behaviour. A study of decision-making Processes in Administrative organisations. Macmillan; 1947

Stanovich K. Rationality and the reflective mind. Oxford University Press; 2010.

Stanovich KE. Rationality and the reflective mind. Oxford University Press; 2011.

Stanovich KE, West RF. On the relative independence of thinking biases and cognitive ability. J Pers Soc Psychol. 2008;94(4):672–95. https://doi.org/10.1037/0022-3514.94.4.672.

Walker M. Why we sleep: the new science of sleep and dreams. Allen Lane; 2017.

Williams. Williams pit stop expertise to help save newborn babies; 2016.

Wilson TD, Brekke N. Mental contamination and mental correction: unwanted influences on judgments and evaluations. Psychol Bull. 1994;116(1):117–42. https://doi.org/10.1037/0033-2909.116.1.117.

Chapter 9
Personality—What Can We Learn from Ourselves and Others?

Don't do an Icarus- Confidence gives you wings but Insight is a great flame retardant."

—Stephen Lash

My blind spots are covered with two eyes.

—Stephen Lash

Faithful are the wounds of a friend but the kisses of an enemy are deceitful.

Proverbs 27 v 6

Abstract Personality may be defined as that which characterises an individual, expressing itself via behaviours, emotions, and thoughts. In this final section I will explore the effect that personality might have on the practice of surgery. Does it influence our choice to even become a surgeon in the first place? Are all the stereotypes accurate, are the jokes justified? Although we cannot change our personality, having insight into how we experience the world and subsequently how we function in it, and further, how others experience us, might offer avenues for improving as surgeons and as members of teams delivering care. I will explore personality through two instruments, Myers-Briggs Type Indicator (MBTI) and the 5 Factor model of personality (The Big 5). As part of this chapter, I asked all my previous fellows to complete the two tests explored and I am thankful that most replied and agreed. Would knowing their personality profiles have allowed a more personalised approach to their training? Could I predict their approach to surgery from their personality? I also reveal my own profile and reflect on how aspects of my personality both help and hinder me.

Keywords Surgical personality · Surgery · Myers briggs type indicator (MBTI) · The Big 5 · Surgeon selection · Surgeon's performance · Surgical decision-making · Surgery improvement · Patient outcome

9.1   Introduction

Personality may be defined as that which characterises an individual, expressing itself via behaviours, emotions, and thoughts. Personality is both innate and acquired, with twin studies demonstrating that heritability can explain about 50% of variance in character traits (Bouchard and McGue 2003; Jang et al. 1996). In this final section I will explore the effect that personality might have on the practice of surgery. I approach this final chapter with excitement and enthusiasm, I feel that personality should make a big difference in how we practise surgery. Does it influence our choice to even become a surgeon in the first place? Are all the stereotypes accurate, are the jokes justified? Although we cannot change our personality, having insight into how we experience the world and subsequently how we function in it, and further, how others experience us, might offer avenues for improving as surgeons and as members of teams delivering care. I will explore personality through two instruments, Myers-Briggs Type Indicator (MBTI) and the 5 Factor model of personality (The Big 5). I am interested in several questions that may arise. Is there a 'surgical personality' and if so, do I have it? This would be reassuring at least! We have all enjoyed, been the butt of, or even enjoyed being the butt of the 'in jokes' around surgeons but how true is it all? If it is true, does the stereotype suggested confer advantage to the practice of surgery? However, personality is never a one-way street and with the advantages must come disadvantages, blind spots and a 'shadow self' to contend with. How might personality affect training both as trainers and as trainees? As part of this chapter, I asked all my previous fellows to complete the two tests explored and I am thankful that most replied and agreed. Would knowing their personality profiles have allowed a more personalised approach to their training? Could I predict their approach to surgery from their personality? I also reveal my own profiles and reflect on how aspects of my personality both help and hinder me.

9.2   The 5 Factor Model of Personality

The journey into personality started with 4500 adjectives proposed by Sir Francis Galton in the late nineteenth century in his work 'Measurements of Character'. He believed these were descriptive of observable and relatively permanent personality traits. Since then, a series of refinements have occurred reducing the number of descriptors and forming terms into clusters. The familiar terms 'Extraversion' and 'neuroticism' were coined by Hans Eysenck in 1947 (Eysenck 1947). Over the 1960s, Cattell narrowed terms down and produced her 16 PF instrument allowing self-assessment. In the late 1960s, 5 global factors, derived from the 16 factors, were identified as; Extraversion, independence, Anxiety, Self-Control and Tough mindedness. The 1970s led to a change in the Zeitgeist surrounding personality with much scepticism regarding predicting behaviour from such personality instruments and the subject fell out of favour. The 1980s and 1990s led to a resurgence of interest in the study of personality. These decades saw the emergence of 'Charismatic leadership' with figures such as Branson and Sugar. The Five Factor model I will use subsequently emerged consisting of Openness, Conscientiousness, Extraversion, Agreeableness and Neuroticism (OCEAN). I would highly recommend the reader take the test in order to further understand and personalise this chapter. There are several online resources available and official websites which offer a more thorough and accurate assessment at a cost.

9.3 Openness

Openness to experience is a general appreciation for art, adventure, ideas, imagination, curiosity and emotion. People who are high on openness are willing to try new things, they are more creative and more aware of their feelings than others and are intellectually curious and keen to self-actualise. They prefer novelty to routine. High openness may also result in riskier behaviour, including drug taking. Low openness people seek fulfilment through perseverance and duty and are seen as dependable, a safe pair of hands, but can also be perceived as dogmatic, stubborn and closed minded.

9.4 Conscientiousness

High Conscientiousness manifests in a high degree of self-discipline in order to achieve against set standards. It requires regulation of impulses and an ability to delay gratification in pursuit of a goal. Low conscientiousness is associated with flexibility and spontaneity but also a lack of reliability and rather haphazard behaviour. High conscientiousness is second only to intelligence in predicting career success.

9.5 Extraversion

Extraversion is characterised by an interest in breadth of activities as opposed to depth. Energy is drawn from external means by significant interactions with the external world, including people, and is characterised by high degree of enthusiasm and action. As a result, extroverts tend to have high visibility in group situations and may appear more dominant. Introverts have lower social engagement energies than extroverts and tend to draw energy from solitude hence the need for more time alone in comparison to extraverts. Introverts are often wrongly assumed to be shy or depressed. Susan Cain would argue that the current work environment favours extraverted leadership but that the tide may be turning in favour of introverted leadership and a move away from extravert dominated decision-making tools. For example, the much utilised 'brainstorming' favours extraverts not necessarily good strategies (Cain 2013).

9.6   Agreeableness

Agreeable individuals value harmony in group situations and value getting along with others. They are generally kind and considerate, trusting and trustworthy, helpful and willing to compromise their interests for the sake of others. They are optimistic about human nature. Alternatively, disagreeable individuals place self-interest above getting along with others, they are less likely to extend themselves in the service of others and are often sceptical about others' motives. They can come across as suspicious, unfriendly and argumentative. I suspect agreeable persons may make excellent transformational leaders and disagreeable leaders may make excellent transactional leaders especially in turnaround scenarios. Agreeableness tends to be higher in women compared to men.

9.7   Neuroticism

Neuroticism is the tendency to experience negative emotions such as anger, anxiety or depression. It is associated with a low tolerance for stress and individuals with high levels of neuroticism are more likely to interpret ordinary situations as threatening. They are more likely to be pessimistic and suffer higher levels of stress at work. This can interfere with making decisions and thinking clearly. Individuals with low levels of neuroticism are less easily upset and less emotionally reactive. They are more calm and emotionally stable and have less negative emotions. Neuroticism tends to be higher in women compared to men.

9.8   The Surgical Personality—What Do You Think?

Having read the above, what would *you* think might form a 'surgical personality', if it exists, and why? I would suggest high conscientiousness and low neuroticism would be of immediate and significant benefit but the remainder perhaps less so. High conscientiousness would result in the relentless pursuit of perfection. Low neuroticism would prevent 'paralysis by analysis' during surgery and reduce levels of stress at times of pressure. This would also be very reassuring for patients and staff alike but especially the surgical trainees being trained if we think back to the Catastrophe model in 'Part I'. However high conscientiousness might also result in self-critical behaviour and a high pressure to perform and low neuroticism might result in more risk-taking behaviour? Low agreeableness might favour progression in very competitive environments (such as surgery) as self-progress is prioritised over getting along with colleagues however, high agreeableness might result in better patient-doctor relationships and better team relationships all essential in delivering excellent healthcare. Extraversion is almost a caricature that has self-perpetuated through urban myth and humour mostly aimed at Orthopaedic surgeons, which I think they like very much. Extraversion might favour progression through apprenticeship models where extended interactions with the Consultant and 'firm' are required, although this model has been largely and rapidly replaced in modern surgical training in favour of competences and box ticking exercises, perhaps favouring introverts. High openness may favour the surgical innovators, who want to do it differently and low openness favour the surgical practitioners who want to do it the same every time. Low openness individuals might resonate with the ideas in 'Lean' surgery however, high openness individuals might experience dissonance in this regard. In short, I am not sure!

9.9 The Surgical Personality the Big 5—What Do the Studies Say?

Studies have analysed the personality types within various fields of medicine and also compared surgeons to the general population. They have found statistically significant variations in personality profiles between surgeons and non-surgeons although these tend to be small samples within single institutions. Whitaker et al. reported an analysis based on survey data of 600 members of the Royal College of Surgeons of England and on a large-scale, UK wide survey, conducted by the BBC on over 385,000 people representing the general public (Whitaker 2018). They used a standard questionnaire consisting of 50 questions from the Five Factor personality assessment and sent it to 20,500 members of the Royal college of Surgeons England. 848 responses (4%) were received which perhaps demonstrates a degree of scepticism as to the usefulness of such research. The final sample consisted of 599 responses, 341 from men and 256 from women. Women make up 15% of surgical specialities on the GMC specialist register (GMC 2022). The BBC Survey relied on traffic to the website rather than active invitations as in the GMC survey. The results demonstrated statistically significant variations in the mean levels of agreeableness, conscientiousness, neuroticism and openness between the surgical and non-surgical populations (Whitaker 2018). Surgeons were more likely to score higher on agreeableness, conscientiousness, neuroticism and openness, with no significant difference in terms of extraversion. Women tended to score much higher on extraversion than men in the surgical population and lower in extroversion than the men in the non-surgical group. The BBC survey found that, with age, people tended to become more agreeable, more conscientious, less open to experience, less neurotic and less extroverted. Whitaker found that older surgeons appear to change as per the general population with the exception of neuroticism, which increased. Older surgeons appear to be more prone to neuroticism than younger surgeons (Whitaker 2018). I felt this was somewhat counterintuitive, the older more experienced surgeon who has seen it all before should surely be less neurotic. However, having read Henry Marsh in his book 'Admissions', he indeed expresses just such a transition (Marsh 2017). This paper seems to disagree with my initial thoughts that surgeons would score low on neuroticism.

In another paper, Sier et al. also explored the surgical personality reviewing multiple Anglo-Saxon studies comparing surgeons to the general population and this included the Whittaker study above which they described as 'incongruent' (Sier et al. 2023). Some English and American studies found that surgeons scored lower on openness and neuroticism but higher on conscientiousness and extraversion compared to the general population (Drosdeck et al. 2015; Hoffman et al. 2010). The largest study on the surgical personality they reviewed was performed on European and Canadian medical students, surgical and non-surgical residents and specialists (Stienen et al. 2018). When comparing physicians and surgeons they found that surgeons scored higher on extraversion ($p = 0.003$) and openness to experience ($p = 0.002$), but lower on neuroticism ($p < 0.001$). There was no difference in agreeableness and conscientiousness (Stienen et al. 2018). Reviewing several Scandinavian studies the differences in Neuroticism were confirmed but also lower agreeableness and higher conscientiousness (Bexelius et al. 2016; Mullola et al. 2018). They also reviewed an American and a Jordanian paper, both finding that conscientiousness and extraversion were higher in the surgical populations with low neuroticism only found in the Jordanian paper (Drosdeck et al. 2015; Nawaiseh et al. 2020). The American study also showed lower scores in agreeableness perhaps indicating cultural differences. The review also included studies looking at the performance of surgical residents attempting to assess suitability and well-being. A study from Texas reviewed the performance of 34 surgical residents in relation to conventional selection measures and the big Five domain scores (Hughes et al. 2019). This study classified participants into 'low performing' and 'non-low performing' residents. They found statistically significant differences in the 'non-low performing' group in terms of higher extroversion, conscientiousness and emotional stability (low neuroticism) as compared to the 'low performing' residents (Hughes et al. 2019). In terms of job satisfaction a study on over 400 trauma surgeons found that the more extroverted and emotionally stable (low neuroticism) surgeons demonstrated higher job satisfaction (Foulkrod et al. 2010). In terms of high levels of patient satisfaction and a positive recommendation of the operating surgeon, high emotional stability (low neuroticism) was significantly associated (Lanz et al. 2018). Burnout was found to be higher in surgeons with high neuroticism and extroversion was protective (Prins et al. 2019).

In summary, the most consistent findings are high levels of conscientiousness, extraversion and low levels of neuroticism with a slight tendency towards high agreeableness and high openness. Low neuroticism seems significant in terms of protecting against burnout, increasing job satisfaction and increasing surgeon recommendation to others by staff and patients. So how do these findings compare to my fellows? (Table 9.1).

Table 9.1 Big 5 results

	Extroversion	Conscientiousness	Neuroticism	Agreeableness	Openness
Me	98	90	34	32	17
Fellow 1	25	56	67	57	8
Fellow 2	50	91	7	71	21
Fellow 3	43	88	39	15	1
Fellow 4	92	83	4	77	75
Fellow 5	20	23	76	50	45
Fellow 6	94	78	44	82	61
Fellow 7	12	85	53	65	18
Fellow 8	43	59	16	80	49
Fellow 9	94	85	18	0	20
Fellow 10	89	96	7	68	35
Average	56	74	33	56	35

The results do reflect the current research findings with high conscientiousness and low neuroticism common at the 74th and 33rd percentiles respectively. There is a tendency towards agreeableness (56th percentile) and extroversion (56th percentile) as in the literature. However, openness was low (35th percentile) in contrast to the research. I have not had the opportunity to train any female fellows to date. We must of course be aware of the law of small numbers and this review was more for interest and analysis than proving a surgical personality.

9.10 Conscientiousness (74th Percentile)

With an average of the 74th percentile, this was universally high except one fellow who bucked the trend with low conscientiousness (and high neuroticism) and yet he was an excellent surgeon, keen to learn and not overly anxious. Without his score the average goes up to the 80th percentile.

9.11 Neuroticism (33rd Percentile)

With an average of the 33rd percentile, this was low. This is the metric I am most fascinated with. As a junior it was always preferable to be trained by a non-anxious presence in the room! If we think back to the Catastrophe model in 'Part I', reducing cognitive anxiety does improve performance and prevents the catastrophic collapse. As a trainee you can bask in the excess confidence in the room and, even more so, borrow it! I have only very rarely come across a level of neuroticism that I felt was not consistent with a surgical career and as far as I am aware they are no longer surgical although I did not formally assess them. Looking over my fellows there were three very low scores but I would not classify any of them as risk takers although they were all at very different stages in their training. My concern, in the introduction, that risk-taking behaviour may be a factor in people with very low neuroticism is not true among my previous fellows, there is much more going on. Likewise, there were two scoring quite high, both at different stages. One certainly expressed a degree of anxiety when being watched and has handed over cases to me when I felt he was more than capable, but he was a good surgeon. The other did struggle somewhat with retinal surface peeling which you can imagine requires very fine motor control, and further is performed under high magnification and watched by all in theatre. I am sure you agree, a situation bound to increase adrenaline and tremor especially as he was very early in his training. The one fellow I would have guessed would be high in neuroticism was in fact middle of the group and scored around the average. It may be other factors are moderating an apparent anxiety be it introversion and a quiet demeanour or very high conscientiousness with very high standards demanded or simply, competence as a result of stage of training which is quite appropriate.

9.12 Extraversion (56th Percentile)

With my fellows, this did not influence surgical ability at whatever stage the trainee was at. It did have an effect on teamwork and integrating with the team in multiple dimensions. Extroverts tended to have a more difficult time being accepted by the team of nurses in theatre. The VR Fellow is always seen to be 'bringing in more work' due to the emergency nature of the speciality but this plus extraversion seemed too much for some of the nurses who, in reality, are already stretched within the NHS. However, they all settled over the year with excellent relationships with staff. Perhaps the agreeableness won over in the end! The introverts were generally more accepted initially and even mothered to some degree. I think extroversion can come across as overconfidence and I am fairly sure that is how I came across during my training. As a trainer I am used to the introvert taking time to process an excellent answer and extroverts coming out with genius and folly in equal measure as they externally process. I do this all the time.

9.13 Agreeableness (56th Percentile)

My fellows score above average in this characteristic (63rd percentile without the outlier). Looking at the outliers the least agreeable trainee was very confident, perhaps the most confident I have trained thus far, and very enthusiastic and not afraid to disagree with me on management. One of the most agreeable fellows had some struggles with certain relationships within the team but he was also very high on extroversion and openness so lots of external processing of constant ideas which included, at times, how to suck eggs.

9.14   Openness (35th Percentile)

My fellows score below average in this characteristic as opposed to the research which found higher levels than average. Looking at the outliers once more, the highest openness fellow frequently wanted to explore other ways of doing things and questioned technique frequently. This often meant challenge and sometimes conflict although they also scored high on extraversion, which would encourage external processing and a degree of talking before thinking, as well as high conscientiousness driving the desire to be better. I really enjoyed working with this fellow. Likewise, the fellow who scored the lowest was a pleasure to work with being very calm and very diligent.

9.15   Conclusions on the Big 5 and Surgery

Knowing the personality of the trainee does not seem to influence how they progressed or how capable they were. Like any relationship there needs to be a degree of flex to get the best out of each other and so appreciating difference can only be a good thing. It is interesting to note that there was a significant degree of agreement with the literature in terms of the major characteristics of surgeons in terms of high conscientiousness and low neuroticism in my fellows. Low neuroticism confers many advantages in terms of job satisfaction, burnout protection and recommendations from former patients and staff. I do not think assessment of the Big 5 has a place in selection because it would have screened out a very good fellow. I think it is in self-reflection that personality is of real use rather than making judgements or assessments about others.

As an extrovert I talk and bring energy to theatre which can manifest as banter and fun but it can be a bit much for some people at times and I have also given difficult feedback in environments I should not have done. High conscientiousness means I am desperate to improve and get better and hope to see this commitment in my trainees so I can be hard on myself and them at times. I have sink or swim enthusiasm. Be enthusiastic with me and I will walk over glass for you, show disinterest and I am gone, there is no in between. I do not quite get my identity from being a surgeon but it is close and my level of conscientiousness can result in a difficulty with criticism. With my low neuroticism, I tend not to worry and this can get me into trouble as I stated earlier in my case where I should have engaged System 2 thinking however, it has also resulted in me embarking on several learning curves as a consultant which have increased my interest and enjoyment of surgery. I generally get good feedback from trainees in theatre and this is likely the result of my low levels of neuroticism but I can also be a harsh critic if enthusiasm is low or an external locus of control is manifest- a particular trigger of mine! I am an early adopter but not an innovator but that's ok, I am low in openness. I want to do it the same way (the best way) every time and this breeds efficiency and a draw towards 'Lean' surgery.

9.16   Big 5 to Try

What are your big 5?
   Do they resonate in general?
   Do they resonate surgically?
   Where might each influence you in a positive and negative direction both in terms of the practice of surgery and in training surgery?
   Can you do anything about this?
   Dare you explore your blind spots by asking others their perceptions of you?
   Can you think back over relationships in theatre through this lens, can it help to explain the positive and negative situations?

9.17   Myers-Briggs Type Indicator (MBTI)

Myers-Briggs Type indicator (MBTI) is a very popular tool for exploring type and is originally based on the work by Carl Jung from his book psychological types (Jung 1921). The test was developed by a mother and daughter partnership, Katherine Briggs and Isabel Briggs-Myers who took Jung's book and simplified and organised it into four dichotomies. Much of the validating research has been carried out by the Myers-Briggs foundation published in its own Journal, the Journal of Psychological Type. It has received criticism for being 'Pseudoscience' however, I have personally found it a very useful lens through which to view the world from marriage preparation through to my MBA and working in teams. It has been used in many studies regarding personality and choice of career in medicine and surgery and I think it is a worthwhile lens through which to view our subject.

   The Myers-Briggs indicator was created during the second world war in an attempt to help women entering the industrial workforce find suitably 'matched' jobs to their type. In 1956 the indicator changed its name to Myers-Briggs Type Indicator (MBTI). Various Universities came on board to develop the indicator and the third edition was published in 1998. The test is a self-administered questionnaire and the results are presented as a four letter 'Type' based on four dichotomies. The four dichotomies are Extroversion/ Introversion (E/I), Sensing/Intuition (S/N), Thinking/Feeling (T/F) and Judging/Perceiving (J/P). The various combinations result in 16 personality types. My own MBTI is ENTJ for example. I will go briefly through the four categories but to fully engage with MBTI I would recommend you consider taking the test before reading on. There are many available on line or you can take the official full test if you so desire.

9.18   Extroversion (E)/Introversion (I)

This dichotomy refers to attitudes and energy. 'E's are energised by the external world and by action and interaction. They tend to prefer action followed by reflection and they tend to externalise thought processes which can be frustrating for others. They do not do well if too much time is spent alone or inactive. 'I's are energised by solitude and they prefer to reflect and then act. In meetings their silence should not be interpreted as inactivity, inside they are often formulating their opinion in great detail and need time to be allowed to express it. 'Brainstorming' favours the extrovert. This silence can frustrate 'E's if they even stop long enough to become aware of the 'I's in the room. If 'I's spend too much time around others their energy levels can fade and they need to withdraw to recharge. 'E's seek breadth of knowledge whereas 'I's seek depth of knowledge.

9.19   Sensing (S)/Intuition (N)

This dichotomy refers to the information gathering functions and the perceiving functions. 'S's tend to gather information from the physical world, accessed through the five senses. They tend to trust information that is tangible and like to be in the present moment. They like details, data and facts. 'N's tend to feel restricted in the physical world preferring to dream of future possibilities drawing on the underlying principles. 'N's are head in the clouds, 'S's are feet on the ground.

9.20   Thinking (T)/Feeling (F)

This dichotomy describes how people make decisions; these are the judging functions. They are used to make decisions based on the sensing functions. 'T's tend to make decisions that are rational and based on data which makes them more detached, better able to decide based on logic and less concerned with the effect of decisions on others. 'F's tend to come to decisions by empathising, seeking harmony and balance. They seek consensus taking onto account the feelings of others. There is a gender bias with females tending to 'F'.

9.21   Judging (J)/Perceiving (P)

This dichotomy reflects how individuals deal with the outside world. 'J's prefer to be organised and plan interactions with the world, they like schedules and order. 'P's are more spontaneous and flexible in their interactions, they can 'go with the flow'. 'J's are more energised by the start gun and 'P's are more energised by the deadline.

There is a lot more detail and complexity with MBTI which can be useful in coaching and personal development. I will not go into this level of detail; it is surplus to requirement for this chapter and, more importantly, I do not have a sufficient depth of understanding myself! However, with my own type 'ENTJ' useful insights can be uncovered as one digs deeper. If you are an 'ENTJ' the following might resonate!

As an 'ENTJ' I enter situations in life with energy and drive, detest inefficiency, love ideas, dislike details which might slow me down and want to get on with it now, not later. Rather than a single headline with its associated and typical characteristics we can explore beneath the surface and even expose a shadow side. These other characteristics are useful for development. If we represent my personality by a family of four in a car with two adults up front and a child and baby in the back. When my 'dominant function' is in control (Extroverted Thinking), as it is most of the time, it is like the adult driving the car of my life with ease in automatic pilot. It is in System 1. It is focussed on solving life's problems, organising and structuring the environment and accomplishing tasks quickly and efficiently. Apparent inefficiency and problems manifest in my gut as unpleasant feelings that I try to push down. However, this is very likely my auxiliary function or the adult sitting in the passenger seat of my car making gentle and very sensible suggestions. For me this 'auxiliary function' is 'Introverted Intuition'. This will ask questions of the 'dominant function' happily charging ahead to solve problems like, "Is there anything you are missing?" and "What might be the actual consequences of this particular action?". Ignoring the 'auxiliary function' can be problematic. It can lead me to making poor decisions in the name of expediency. It is therefore an area for personal development in order to improve performance and is best accessed in System 2. The 'tertiary function' is the older child sitting in the back seat of the car. For me this is 'Extroverted Sensing' which can manifest in seeking out novel sensations, physical thrills and material comforts. It does not manifest often or with much power as it's in the back seat but an element of surgery satisfies this function for me as does a walk in the woods or a Spa Day. Finally, we have the baby in the back seat and for me this is 'Introverted Feeling' and represents my 'inferior function'. To put a positive spin on the baby, it offers much room for personal development although thankfully it is usually fast asleep! However, when it kicks off it is very unpleasant. 'Introverted feeling' manifests as extremely immature feelings which can be overwhelming. I can suddenly feel 8 years old, fed up and stating that 'I do not want to play anymore and I am taking my ball back!' It's extremely unpleasant and when it continues for months it is described as being 'in the grip'. Being in the grip can look like burnout and having experienced it, it is extremely unpleasant. Thankfully for me it resulted in post-traumatic growth and looking back was very useful. For more information on this deep dive, I would recommend 'Was that really me?' by Naomi Quenk (Quenk 2002). I am in no doubt that understanding yourself is an important step for self-development both in life in general and in surgery specifically.

Having gained a basic understanding of MBTI, I want to look at the evidence in terms of its application to healthcare and specifically surgery. Are certain 'Types' more common in surgery as found with the Big 5?

9.22   The Surgical Personality—What Do You Think?

I would suggest that 'J' is of importance given the order and process required to perform surgery and the need for organising lists, getting them started and keeping them going. All lists want to start late and stop continuously, it's a battle. 'T' might be favourable in getting through the list but might lead to an unpleasant atmosphere in theatre without care and attention. 'S' would favour being in the moment and dealing with feedback through the senses although 'N' might lead to innovation. 'E' might bring energy to a list and enthusiasm; 'I' might bring sense and calm. Again, I don't know.

9.23   The Surgical Personality MBTI—What Do the Studies Say?

In one 2010 study, with a low sample size (39), and looking at trainees who were generation X (1965–1980), the most frequent personality type of the resident surgeon was found to be 'ISTJ' accounting for almost a third of all residents (Swanson et al. 2010) The 'I' Preference contrasted with previous studies suggesting 'E' was more common in surgery. They felt changes in surgical training, with a move away from the apprentice model, might have resulted in the change in personality profile of the trainees. However, there were no significant differences in the other types, 'S/N', 'T/F' or 'J/P' (Swanson et al. 2010). In a specific study of ophthalmologists in 2021, Haider et al. reviewed the profiles of 66 residents (Haidar et al. 2021). The response rate was 48% overall, again a small study. The most significant difference was in the Judging (J)/Perceiving (P) dimension at 67% versus 33% ($p = 0.007$). Trainees were also more likely to be Thinking (T) than Feeling (F) at 64% versus 36% ($p = 0.027$), Extroverted (E) than Introverted (I) at 62% versus 38% ($p = 0.049$). However, Sensing (S) and intuition (N) were not significantly different at 56% versus 44% ($p = 0.325$) (Haidar et al. 2021). They also found that the three most common types were ESTJ, ENTJ and ISTJ at around 13.6% each compared to 11%, 6% and 10% in the general population. Although finding a tendency towards 'E' as opposed to 'I' as in the Swanson study, both found ISTJ to be a common Type (Swanson et al. 2010). They also found similar results to a study on ENT (Ear Nose and Throat to avoid potential confusion!) residents, the most common types were ESTJ and ISTJ (Zardouz et al. 2011). Zardouz also found that 'E' and 'T' types were more likely to pursue a surgical specialty compared to their 'I' and 'F' counterparts. Given the similarities between the two specialities they felt it may be that personalities were attracted to the specific field of medicine rather than being influenced by it. However, they also found some evidence of change in Type over the years of training perhaps suggesting the field might influence the Type. For example, the J/P dichotomy was 50:50 at year 2, 53:47 at Year 3 but 83:17 for graduates (Haidar et al. 2021). This was also seen in two other studies (Contessa et al. 2013; Sliwa and Shade-Zeldow 1994). In another study which looked at various specialities, Chang et al. found, when comparing non-surgical and surgical specialties, the E/I and T/F dimensions were significant in differentiating the two. 'T' preference was more common in the surgical specialities (77.8%) compared to the non-surgical specialties (52.2%). 'E' was more common in the surgical specialities (61%) whereas 'I' was more common in the non-surgical specialities (56–61%). 'S' was similar at 83% for surgical and 78% for non-surgical. Finally, they found that although 'J' was high in all groups it was more common in surgical specialities (78%) compared to non-surgical specialties at (67%) (Chang et al. 2019). Ramachandran et al., extracted quantitative and qualitative data from studies on MBTI in healthcare completed between 1975 and 2018. They reviewed 41 studies out of an initial pool of nearly 700 and categorised findings into one of seven sections ranging from speciality preference, of specific relevance to our discussion, to selection of trainees, evaluation, performance and burnout. They argued that MBTI was a potentially powerful tool for medical education but that of all the studies they reviewed, 30% looked at its role in specialty choice and results were inconsistent (Ramachandran et al. 2020). They found a shift since the 1960s towards 'T' and 'J' in all specialities. They also reviewed studies that indicated a shift in type over the training period with a study by Taylor showing a shift in Family Medicine residents during training. (Taylor et al. 1990) Brown found that fifty-seven percent of medical students change their MBTI preferences between first and fourth years (Brown and Peppler 1994). They suggested that if MBTI was going to be used to help in speciality selection is should be administered just before selection is made (Brown and Peppler 1994). Contessa found that surgeons with E, T and P demonstrated a higher tolerance for risk with I, F and J exhibiting risk aversion, a finding replicated in other studies outside medicine (Contessa et al. 2013).

On reviewing these studies, the findings suggest that 'E' is more common than 'I', 'T' is more common than 'F' and 'J' more common than 'P'. The 'N/S' dichotomy seems less relevant. So how do these findings compare to my fellows? (Table 9.2).

The only finding consistent with the literature was that 'J' predominated. As opposed to a preference for 'T' in the literature, 'F' predominated. The 'F' dominance is also interesting given that I have not trained a female surgeon to date as there is usually a bias towards 'T' in males. These results were based on a shorter online assessment as opposed to the more rigorous and extensive official tests and are based on small numbers so may have errors. Fellow 10 scored 89 on Extraversion on the Big 5 but came out as an 'I' on MBTI. Being forced to choose with MBTI might influence or even change the results as compared to the Big 5. 'S' also predominates

Table 9.2 MBTI results

	E/I	N/S	T/F	P/J
Me	E	N	T	J
Fellow 1	I	S	T	J
Fellow 2	I	S	F	J
Fellow 3	I	S	F	J
Fellow 4	E	N	F	J
Fellow 5	I	S	F	J
Fellow 6	E	S	F	P
Fellow 7	I	S	F	J
Fellow 8	I	N	F	J
Fellow 9	E	S	T	J
Fellow 10	I	N	F	J
	70% I	70% S	80%F	90% J

among my Fellows although the literature found no correlation in this dichotomy. We of course need to be wary of the law of small numbers once more, this is for reflection only!

9.24 Reflections on Results

9.24.1 J/P (90% J)

As in the literature, 'J' predominates at 90%. I would classify our theatre as very much formed in the fashion of 'J' as a result of previous consultants who developed the service over the years and trained me. They placed a high value on efficiency and volume given we only had two theatres. It may be this more pressured environment also suits 'J's. When interviewing for potential fellows we tend to ask a question that probes attitudes to efficiency and running an efficient list as our lists are busy. I suspect we have deliberately, although unknowingly, selected those for whom this is a high value inadvertently favouring 'J's'. Theatre is busy and emergencies are frequent and getting on with the list is essential to avoid constant late finishes. 'J's' will tend to get to the ward early and get prepared and are eager to make progress through the cases. There is a pace and sense of urgency about them. However, like all aspects of personality, there is a downside. Getting through the list for the sake of getting through it can result in patients becoming numbers we need to push through if we are not careful. If we are already likely operating in System 1, which wants to answer more complex questions with simple answers, we are at increased risk of cognitive bias and errors. Less haste more speed. Of all the traits with MBTI, this is the one people who work with me would likely caricature me with. I hate starting late, wasting time, inefficiency and finishing late. I bring a lot of energy to theatre to try to ensure we start on time. I will tell the new fellows that "Time lost at the start of the list is time lost forever!" Some like the pace others find it annoying and disturbing and even, dare I say it 'unsafe'. I disagree. Delaying an urgent case is certainly unsafe and as I explored earlier in 'Part I' with the concept of 'IZOF', I work best with a degree of pace and urgency.

9.25   E/I (70% E)

As in the literature there are more 'E's than 'I's. As I argued before, this dichotomy is more likely to influence the relationships and interactions with the team in theatre rather than the actual practice of surgery although it would not surprise me if the 'E' ends the day energised, the "I" exhausted.

9.26   T/F (80% F)

I had predicted that 'T' would predominate and the literature supported that view however, my fellows were 80% F! I am sure they have significantly contributed to the sense of harmony in our theatre, I am thankful to them all. My speciality has many unplanned and emergency cases and theatres are often busy and change at the last minute. Taking the team with you is a very important skill in delivering safe care and in a pleasant environment. The 'F' is more naturally able to deliver this than the 'T'. As a 'T' I need to control the urge to make progress at any cost. I often fail to do this when I think that people are being obstructive or deliberately inefficient but even more commonly, when additional bureaucracy has been introduced into the processes yet again.

9.27   N/S (70% S)

I had predicted that 'S' would predominate but in fact 'N' did. However, the literature generally finds no pattern in this dichotomy. I would suggest the 'N's' are the innovators and the 'S's' the practitioners and it would be interesting to compare these findings to the Big 5 in terms of Openness with high openness perhaps more likely 'N'? (Although I am low on openness and am an 'N' not an 'S'). Again, I can appreciate both the thought through detailed analysis post-surgery of the 'S' and the ideas of the 'N'. I would argue we need both in surgery. We need to reflect on data and we need to dream of new ways of doing things. As an 'N' I have to discipline myself to prospectively audit to get data and I am grateful for this effort. It has formed an important foundation of my practice but it did not come naturally.

9.28   Conclusion—MBTI

There was agreement with the literature in terms of a preference for surgeons to demonstrate 'J' but in contrast to the literature my fellows were more 'F' as opposed to 'T'. As I reflected on each trainee, their MBTI did not seem to influence how they progressed or how capable they were as surgeons. Given the reduction inherent in MBTI to just 16 types and the dichotomous nature of the results, it does reveal difference more obviously than the Big 5. I would certainly not recommend using it in terms of selection. Once more it may be best used in self-reflection rather than in making judgements of others.

9.29   To Try

Take the MBTI assessment, either the shorter online tests or, for a more accurate result, the official site is preferable.

   Looking at each dimension how does this influence your behaviours and how might people opposite to you behave?

   How might your MBTI influence your surgery for the better and for the worse?

   How might your opposite behave and can you learn from them?

   Where are your development opportunities as a result of your MBTI?

9.30   Comparison Between the Five Factor Model and MBTI

MBTI gives a personality type whereas the Five Factor model gives personality traits. The traits are measured in the five domains and underly aspects of behaviour and are measured along a continuum. MBTI on the other hand results in a dichotomy along four axes with a limited assessment in term of strength, resulting in preferences. These preferences are often likened to handedness in that a right-handed person can write with their left hand but it takes more effort. As such there is no value judgement in the MBTI assessment, 'E' is not better than 'I' for example. In the Five Factor model certain traits are preferred high or low in terms of functioning in the world. For example, high neuroticism is likely to result in negative emotion and susceptibility to depression, not desirable for most people. High openness suggests high creativity and a desire for adventure, including misadventure, whereas low openness may result in rigidity or perhaps more positively, stability. The MBTI can be interpreted in terms of both strengths and weaknesses. Knowing this is of use in working on your 'shadow' side, or your inferior functions and can improve decision making and interaction with others as well as leading to an appreciation of difference. The Five Factor model gives an assessment of individual aspects of personality and is broader based and useful for comparison as opposed to the limited 16 types of MBTI. There is more nuance in the Five Factor model given 5 traits along 5 continuums. The Five Factor model also allows more focussed personal development towards self-actualisation with or without therapy. Although the two tests are different in their approach and measurement there is some interesting overlap between the two discussed in the literature.

In one study, 160 adults completed both tests. The agreeableness score was corre-lated only with the 'T/F' dimension with high agreeableness seen in 'F' type. A high conscientiousness score was correlated with both 'T' and 'J' Types. Extroversion was strongly correlated in both tests whilst the neuroticism score was not related to any MBTI sub-scale score. The openness dimension was correlated with all four but especially with the 'N' type (Furnham 1996). Another study looked at 161 female and 48 Male Canadian students. They also found strong correlation between the extroversion and 'E' type. Openness was again correlated to 'N' and agreeableness with the 'F' type. They also found a correlation with conscientiousness and the 'J' type (MacDonald et al. 1994). Finally, a study by McCrae and Costa found similar correlations among 267 men and 201 women from 19 to 93 years of age. They compared results from MBTI and the Five Factor model of personality as measured by their own personal inventory. In both men and women there was a strong corre-lation between 'E' on MBTI and extroversion on The Five Factor model, 'N' with openness, 'F' with agreeableness and 'J' with conscientiousness (McCrae and Costa 1989).

These observations make intuitive sense in my opinion and are consistent with the findings in my Fellows. A 'J' is likely to get on with tasks quickly and efficiently demonstrating high conscientiousness whereas the 'P' is likely to spend a lot of time thinking and researching and keeping options open until the last minute. My fellows scored very high on conscientiousness and were 90% 'J' in agreement with the findings in the literature. However, once again, the one fellow who scored very low on conscientiousness is the exception as an unexpected 'J'. An 'F' is likely to be concerned with others feeling and gaining consensus hence the correlation with agreeableness. A 'T' wants to get the task completed with logical thinking and little regard to others feelings. My fellows scored high on agreeableness, supported by the literature, but were 80% 'F' whereas the literature suggested 'T' should predominate. An 'N' is likely to be 'open' to new ideas given they prefer to take in information in concepts and like to make connections and think big as opposed to the 'S' who likes to work with information gained through the 5 senses. My fellows scored low on openness and were 70% 'S' which is in agreement with the literature.

9.31   Conclusion

There seems to be a surgical personality. The most consistent findings are high levels of conscientiousness, extraversion and low levels of neuroticism with is a slight tendency towards high agreeableness and high openness. Low neuroticism seems significant in terms of protecting against burnout, increasing job satisfaction and increasing surgeon recommendation to others by staff and patients. On MBTI the 'J' type predominates and this correlates with high conscientiousness, as does the 'T' Type. Low neuroticism has no correlate with the MBTI. A preference for extroversion on the Five Factor model was also found in the MBTI literature with a slight preference for 'E' although the changing structure of surgical education might see introversion ascendant in the coming years as we move away from 'the Firm' towards competencies.

Although there does appear to be a surgical personality and I appear to have it (relief) I have been disappointed with its application especially in terms of its influence on my fellows. Knowing their personality did not help me assess them as surgeons. I think the main benefit of personality is in self-reflection and self-development. I suspect that in the same way basketball players are tall, surgeons have core personality similarities but their expression and outworking in surgical practice is heavily influenced and moderated by a complex mix of the other personality characteristics, experience and intelligence to name but a few.

References

Bexelius TS, Olsson C, Järnbert-Pettersson H, Parmskog M, Ponzer S, Dahlin M. Association between personality traits and future choice of specialisation among Swedish doctors: a cross-sectional study. Postgrad Med J. 2016;92(1090):441–6. https://doi.org/10.1136/postgradmedj-2015-133478.

Bouchard TJ, McGue M. Genetic and environmental influences on human psychological differences. J Neurobiol. 2003;54(1):4–45. https://doi.org/10.1002/neu.10160.

Brown F, Peppler RD. Changes in medical students' Myers-Briggs "preferences" between their first and fourth years of school. Acad Med. 1994;69(3):244. https://doi.org/10.1097/00001888-199403000-00024.

Cain S. Quiet: the power of introverts in a world that can't stop TalkingCain, S. Penguin; 2013.

Chang Y-C, Tseng H-M, Xiao X, Ngerng RYL, Wu, C-L, Chaou C-H (2019) Examining the association of career stage and medical specialty with personality preferences-a cross-sectional survey of junior doctors and attending physicians from various specialties.https://doi.org/10.1186/s12909-019-1789-2

Contessa J, Suarez L, Kyriakides T, Nadzam G. The influence of surgeon personality factors on risk tolerance: a pilot study. J Surg Educ. 2013;70(6):806–12. https://doi.org/10.1016/j.jsurg.2013.07.014.

Drosdeck JM, Osayi SN, Peterson LA, Yu L, Ellison EC, Muscarella P. Surgeon and nonsurgeon personalities at different career points. J Surg Res. 2015;196(1):60–6. https://doi.org/10.1016/j.jss.2015.02.021.

Eysenck HJ (1947) Dimensions of personality. K. Paul, Trench, Trubner.

Foulkrod KH, Field C, Brown CVR. Trauma surgeon personality and job satisfaction: results from a national survey. Am Surg. 2010;76(4):422–7. https://doi.org/10.1177/000313481007600422.

Furnham A. The big five versus the big four: the relationship between the Myers-Briggs Type Indicator (MBTI) and NEO-PI five factor model of personality. Personality Individ Differ. 1996;21(2):303–7. https://doi.org/10.1016/0191-8869(96)00033-5.

GMC. The Workforce report 2022. The state of medical education and practice in the UK 2022. www.Gmc-Uk.Org/Workforce2022.

Haidar M, Ridha F, Ling J, Akhter M, Kueny L, Sabbagh O, Kim C, Chin Loy K. Myers-Briggs type indicator personality types of ophthalmology residents. J Academ Ophthal. 2021;13(02):e158–62. https://doi.org/10.1055/s-0041-1732346.

Hoffman BM, Coons MJ, Kuo PC. Personality differences between surgery residents, nonsurgery residents, and medical students. Surgery. 2010;148(2):187–93. https://doi.org/10.1016/j.surg.2010.04.005.

Hughes BD, Perone JA, Cummins CB, Sommerhalder C, Tyler DS, Bowen-Jallow KA, Radhakrishnan RS. Personality testing may identify applicants who will become successful in general surgery residency. J Surg Res. 2019;233:240–8. https://doi.org/10.1016/j.jss.2018.08.003.

Jang KL, Livesley WJ, Vernon PA. Heritability of the big five personality dimensions and their facets: a twin study. J Pers. 1996;64(3):577–92. https://doi.org/10.1111/j.1467-6494.1996.tb00522.x.

Jung CG. Psychologische typen. Rascher Verlag; 1921

Lanz JJ, Gregory PJ, Menendez ME, Harmon L. Dr. Congeniality: Understanding the Importance of Surgeons' Nontechnical Skills Through 360° Feedback. J Surg Educat 2018;75(4), 984–92. https://doi.org/10.1016/j.jsurg.2017.12.006

MacDonald DA, Anderson PE, Tsagarakis CI, Holland CJ. Examination of the relationship between the Myers-Briggs type indicator and the neo personality inventory. Psychol Rep. 1994;74(1):339–44. https://doi.org/10.2466/pr0.1994.74.1.339.

McCrae RR, Costa PT. Reinterpreting the Myers-Briggs type indicator from the perspective of the five-factor model of personality. J Pers. 1989;57(1):17–40. https://doi.org/10.1111/j.1467-6494.1989.tb00759.x.

Mullola S, Hakulinen C, Presseau J, Ruiz G, de Porras D, Jokela M, Hintsa T, Elovainio M. Personality traits and career choices among physicians in Finland: employment sector, clinical patient contact, specialty and change of specialty. BMC Med Educ. 2018;18(1):52. https://doi.org/10.1186/s12909-018-1155-9.

Nawaiseh M, Haddadin R, Al Droubi B, Nawaiseh H, Alarood S, Aborajooh E, Abufaraj M, Abu-Yaghi N. The association between personality traits and specialty preference among medical students in Jordan. Psychol Res Behav Manag. 2020;13:599–607. https://doi.org/10.2147/PRBM.S262062.

Prins DJ, van Vendeloo SN, Brand PLP, Van der Velpen I, de Jong K, van den Heijkant F, Van der Heijden FMMA, Prins JT. The relationship between burnout, personality traits, and medical specialty. A national study among Dutch residents. Medical Teacher, 2019;41(5), 584–590. https://doi.org/10.1080/0142159X.2018.1514459.

Quenk NL. Was that really me? Davies-Black Publishing; 2002

Ramachandran V, Loya A, Shah KP, Goyal S, Hansoti EA, Caruso AC. Myers-Briggs type indicator in medical education: a narrative review and analysis. Health Professions Education. 2020;6(1):31–46. https://doi.org/10.1016/j.hpe.2019.03.002.

Sier VQ, Schmitz RF, Schepers A, van der Vorst JR. Exploring the surgical personality. The Surgeon. 2023;21(1):1–7. https://doi.org/10.1016/j.surge.2022.01.008.

Sliwa JA, Shade-Zeldow Y. Physician personality types in physical medicine and rehabilitation as measured by the Myers-Briggs type indicator. Am J Phys Med Rehabil. 1994;73(5):308–12. https://doi.org/10.1097/00002060-199409000-00002.

Stienen MN, Scholtes F, Samuel R, Weil A, Weyerbrock A, Surbeck W. Different but similar: personality traits of surgeons and internists—results of a cross-sectional observational study. BMJ Open. 2018;8(7): e021310. https://doi.org/10.1136/bmjopen-2017-021310.

Swanson JA, Antonoff MB, D'Cunha J, Maddaus MA. Personality profiling of the modern surgical trainee: insights into generation X. J Surg Educ. 2010;67(6):417–20. https://doi.org/10.1016/J.JSURG.2010.07.017.

Taylor AD, Clark C, Sinclair AE. Personality types of family practice residents in the 1980s. Acad Med. 1990;65(3):216–8. https://doi.org/10.1097/00001888-199003000-00018.

Whitaker M. The surgical personality: does it exist? The Annals of the Royal College of Surgeons of England. 2018;100(1):72–7. https://doi.org/10.1308/rcsann.2017.0200.

Zardouz S, German MA, Wu EC, Djalilian HR. Personality types of otolaryngology resident applicants as described by the Myers-Briggs type indicator. Otolaryngology-Head and Neck Surgery. 2011;144(5):714–8. https://doi.org/10.1177/0194599810397793.

Conclusion—What Have We Learned?

I have really enjoyed exploring surgery in 'three boxes' through these three 'Parts' and I hope you have learned as much as I have. It is clear that *'They have good hands'* is entirely insufficient when it comes to describing a good surgeon. Focussing on improving those hands will be of limited benefit in the pursuit of excellence. It is complex and there is no magic trick, app or life hack. It is about slow deliberate formation in the direction of 'virtuosity' and every surgery, every surgical decision and manoeuvre will help or hinder you in your quest.

I hope I have demonstrated how the boxes over lap and influence one another. For example, from Part I I can take home several of the techniques from Sports Psychology, specifically imagery and goal setting and apply these to the Lean approach to surgery from Part II. This feels very comfortable and natural for me as a 'J' and 'T' on MBTI and my high conscientiousness and low openness on the Big 5 from Part III. Further I can apply the micro technique from Part I and lean in Part II and apply it to several realms, from post-surgery review and audit in Parts II and III, exposing heuristics and cognitive bias and challenging System 1 in Part III, to embracing and learning from failure back in Part II. You may well have taken very different lessons and perspectives away as might your trainee/boss, enjoy discussing them over coffee.

These are of course limited perspectives and there are others. For example, try reading the book as a patient. What is of value to you now as you read each part? What remains relevant but what becomes irrelevant and why? What is your motivation in becoming a surgeon or practicing as a surgeon and how does this influence your reading of the book? Does Lean offer increased productivity, increased profitability or simply increased kudos?

I hope that in reading this book, in owning a copy with scribbles in the margins and coffee stains on the pages acquired during robust and diverse post-surgery discussions with colleagues that go well beyond your 'hands', you can venture into territory well beyond my limited perspectives, away from the concrete, the boardwalks, the sands and the shallows into the deep! Have fun!

© The Editor(s) (if applicable) and The Author(s), under exclusive license
to Springer Nature Switzerland AG 2024
S. Lash, *Improving Surgical Skills and Outcomes*,
https://doi.org/10.1007/978-3-031-66690-2

Index